What healthcare providers are saying about *Surviving American Healthcare*:

Val Conrad's *Surviving American Healthcare* contains information every patient should know and guides readers toward getting the most from their healthcare experience in a way that is easy to read and understand. As an ICU nurse, I know how overwhelming hospitalization and dealing with the healthcare system can be, for both patients and their families. I would recommend this book to everyone to help them cope and understand both their rights, and what they can do to help healthcare workers maximize the quality of their experience.

– Danny Dunaway, RN, University of Mississippi Medical Center MICU

Surviving American Healthcare will help patients and their loved ones understand how gaining a better knowledge of a patient's medical problems can help to get more effective healthcare.

–Emmett Martin, EMT-Paramedic, (retired)

SURVIVING AMERICAN HEALTHCARE

ADVOCATING FOR YOURSELF OR SOMEONE YOU LOVE

Valerie Conrad, BS, BSN, RN

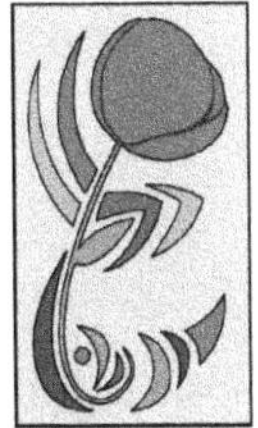

Praeclarus Press, LLC

www.PraeclarusPress.com

Praeclarus Press, LLC
2504 Sweetgum Lane
Amarillo, Texas 79124 USA
806-553-5855
www.PraeclarusPress.com

DISCLAIMER

The information contained in this publication is advisory only and is not intended to replace sound clinical judgment or individualized patient care. The author disclaims all warranties, whether expressed or implied, including any warranty as the quality, accuracy, safety, or suitability of this information for any particular purpose.

ISBN: 978-0-9854180-1-4
ISBN (Kindle version): 978-0-9854180-3-8
ISBN (Nook version): 978-0-9854180-4-5

Cover Design: Ken Tackett

Developmental Editing: Kathleen Kendall-Tackett

Copy Editing: Diana Cassar-Uhl

Layout & Design: Todd Rollison

Illustrations: Cary Raulston.

TABLE OF CONTENTS

SECTION II
WHEN YOU ARE ILL

SECTION IV
MEDICATIONS

SECTION V
APPENDICES

FOREWORD

Surviving American Healthcare offers a fresh, timely perspective of how each of us can successfully navigate today's confusing healthcare system by providing us with an informative and detailed guide covering topics such as knowing what is important to communicate (and how to communicate) with your healthcare provider, as well as a comprehensive primer on medications. Other helpful topics include advanced directives, and an overview of the healthcare reform law.

As a result of her unique experiences in healthcare, Val Conrad offers clear explanations of the most realistic ways to better one's experience as a patient or as a family member of a patient who needs a well-informed advocate. I highly recommend it be used as a reference by anyone who is a patient or loves a patient.

Deborah Davenport, Ph.D., RN
Associate Professor of Nursing
College of Nursing and Health Sciences
West Texas A&M University

PREFACE

The American healthcare system can be difficult to navigate—even for healthcare professionals. But knowing how to do it can mean the difference between good care and care that is sub-par. In some cases, it can mean the difference between life and death. I know this from both personal experience and from the decades I've spent as a healthcare provider. I've been a paramedic and am now a nurse in an intensive care unit. I'm the daughter of parents who suffered through the healthcare system, and I have been a patient myself.

Healthcare providers themselves don't intend to make healthcare complex. Part of the issue is cost. Insurance companies and multi-million-dollar lawsuits have complicated the picture, and the outcomes often have little to do with the actual care of patients. Ideally, medicine should not be about making a profit. It should be about providing the best medical care to the most people—but that might mean that providers do not even cover their costs.

Triage is a word that we associate with mass-casualty disasters, sorting and prioritizing patients and resources to increase the chances of recovery of the most people, knowing that some may not survive. Unfortunately, providers cannot save every patient, and some patients do not want to be saved. I'm not saying that we should not try to save every patient, but sometimes healthcare providers try to save patients who have very little chance of survival. Success is not measured by the end result of a beating heart and breathing lungs. Resources are better focused on saving patients who have a life with quality, not just existence.

In the end, healthcare providers must evaluate the care of each patient by this single question:

Did we do right by the patient?

"Doing right" means we did everything we could to elicit the best possible outcome. However, doing right might occasionally mean that the patient does not live. We need to remember that all of us will die eventually, and there are times when being "alive" is worse than being allowed to die with dignity and peace.

These are hard decisions to make, and for me, they are not merely theoretical. In 2009, my father suffered a sudden cardiac arrest. He simply dropped to the floor at a grocery store. The ambulance was nearby, and the code (as those who work a cardiac arrest call it) lasted over twenty minutes before my father's pulse returned. From a small town, he was flown to a larger hospital, spent two days on a ventilator, 15 days in the cardiac care unit, and 10 more in a rehab unit to rebuild his strength. He survived and was able to live independently at home for the next 18 months. His recovery was pretty incredible, given his age and past cardiac history. Even so, my sister and I had to fight the healthcare system over many issues in both the hospital and the rehab facility. A medical school resident let a jugular-vein intravenous catheter insertion guide wire slip into my father's chest. In the cardiac care unit (CCU), my father began to hallucinate, probably due to a combination of sleep deprivation and morphine, even in appropriate dosages. Once he was awake, he refused to eat poultry, but it continued to arrive on his mealtime plate. We ultimately had to say he was allergic to chicken and turkey so that his meals no longer included those meats. There were many other issues, all of which demonstrated to me that a patient needs to have an advocate, someone to fight when he cannot do so himself.

Months after my father's cardiac-arrest survival, his cardiologist wanted to change his pacemaker to a combination pacer and internal defibrillator that would provide a shock in the event he had another episode of the same fatal dysrhythmia. My father said no, that he did not want to survive another "episode" if it meant losing even the same small amount of quality of life he'd lost the first time his heart stopped. The first arrest took about 10% of his abilities, and he did not want to face possibly losing an additional 20%—or more—of his functioning.

As his daughter, I didn't want to support that decision, but as his advocate, I understood why my father felt that way, and I rallied his decision when his doctors offered other treatments he did not want. Honestly, it broke my heart to see him write his do-not-resuscitate orders for outside the hospital, but I carried them with me in case I needed to produce them.

You may face a similar scenario, either as a patient or someone who loves one. Even in more routine matters, you need to educate yourself. You need to understand the facts about your health, any conditions you may have, and your treatment options. In addition, you need to understand your rights, and then stand up for the decisions you make. This can be difficult, but it is absolutely necessary. Exercising your rights may also mean saying "no" to tests, vaccines, medications, or procedures where the benefit does not justify the risk, or where treatment will not provide a cure or comfort. If you are faced with a serious illness, you need an advocate to speak for you when you cannot. My goal is to aid you in this process. With that in mind, this book strives to help you be responsible for your own health by:

- Expecting reasonable medical outcomes of care,
- Knowing about diseases and conditions you may have,
- Understanding your medications and possible drug interactions,
- Making advocacy a personal advantage, and
- Actively participating in the care you receive.

I offer to you, patients and loved ones alike, a guide to being a better patient, standing up for your rights, gaining understanding of your health, and making difficult choices with knowledge beforehand. We can't afford to let the healthcare system make our decisions by default. Being prepared is the biggest step any of us can take to stay healthy—and to survive American healthcare.

SECTION I

YOU IN THE HEALTHCARE SYSTEM

CHAPTER 1

Introduction

American healthcare provides some of the most advanced assessment and treatment in the world, but the foundation on which our medical system was built has begun to fail. Exorbitant costs, limited coverage, lack of insurance portability, abuse of billing and social services, and uncontrolled errors have made accessing and receiving quality healthcare difficult, with or without health insurance.

In March 2010, President Barack Obama signed into law the Patient Protection and Affordable Care Act, putting into motion a decade of changes and improvements to the existing system. In June 2012, the U.S. Supreme Court upheld the constitutionality of the law (see Appendix C). Very few Americans dispute that healthcare needs to be improved, but most agree that reform shouldn't take thousands of pages to accomplish. I've read it, though I wonder how many people who voted the bill into law did. It offers some very necessary corrections to healthcare's biggest weaknesses, but it is vague and convoluted—legal verbiage at its finest.

No matter what changes in healthcare lay ahead, your best defense is to participate fully in your own care, and to educate yourself so that you can make informed decisions. Whether you are a patient, or someone who cares for one, knowledge is power—and that power cannot be taken away.

Taking Charge of Your Health

The first step to taking charge of your health is to know all you can about any conditions or diseases you might have. In many cases, the terms *disease, condition, disorder*, and *illness* are used interchangeably, but they are not always the same thing. There is an obvious difference in diseases that can be cured compared to those that require lifetime management, such as the flu versus diabetes. Contagious diseases are also separated from those that are not communicable, as well as those that have a genetic link. Knowing the nature of your medical condition will help you make decisions for yourself and those around you. While protecting infants or children from your cold or flu is a simple matter of space, time, and basic hygiene, protecting those around you from a chronic communicable disease, such as hepatitis, requires a vastly different approach. Young adults who carry a gene for an incurable condition such as Huntington's disease may choose to not have children who could have a 25% chance of having the disease. (Huntington's is a neurodegenerative disorder that leads to cognitive decline and jerky body movements.)

Regardless of the cause or communicability, your diseases and conditions affect you and the people in your life. Treatments can be brief or lifelong. Understanding what those treatments are, the expected results, and your alternatives will allow you to successfully participate in the preventive care and treatment you receive.

Personally and professionally, I have seen how patient knowledge and participation can directly impact the care received from healthcare providers and facilities. Being involved doesn't always guarantee better care, but knowledge of how a disease is assessed and treated shows your interest in the outcome. Ultimately, you are responsible for your health and management of your illnesses. You may have options in the type of care you receive, including advanced directives, organ donation, and hospice care. Understanding these options before a medical crisis makes deciding about them much easier.

Negotiating the Obstacles to Good Care

Medicine has become complicated in the twenty-first century. Patients born before the 1960s grew up in a time when doctors were immortal, always correct, and never questioned. In contrast, the advent of the Internet makes many younger patients willing to question, and sometimes challenge, the authority of a physician, especially after doing research on their own. They may demand different tests or second opinions. Still, there are patients in between, who have neither the knowledge nor confidence to investigate their own health issues. These patients need an advocate who can help them make decisions.

Another issue is that some patients will not interact with healthcare providers when there is an age or gender difference. A patient might prefer an older doctor with more experience, or a man might not wish to see a female doctor. In emergencies, and in rural settings, a patient may abstain from medical care rather than accept care from someone too young or of the "wrong" gender. These barriers need to be resolved for the patient's best interests in all medical care.

Get the Information You Need

Information can be a double-edged sword, but it is essential to receiving good care. While there are many good health websites with accurate information, there are also many with wrong or misleading information. To further complicate matters, some pharmaceutical companies market directly to consumers via television and print media, encouraging patients to ask for specific (and often more expensive) name-brand medications. Patients may go for doctor appointments, demanding a prescription for something they've seen on television or in a magazine, in some cases without medical evidence that they suffer from the condition for which the drug is given. There are herbs and supplements that are not FDA approved or regulated at all, and come with fine-print disclosure:

> This statement has not been evaluated by the Food and Drug Administration. This product is not intended to diagnose, treat, cure, or prevent any disease.

Lawyers may also create confusion by advertising directly to consumers for the express purpose of enrolling them in class-action lawsuits filed against manufacturers for drug effects and equipment failures. Be particularly leery of these. Some claims are legitimate, and others are not. You are probably better off seeking legal counsel closer to home than hiring someone through a television advertisement.

Obtaining good information may be a challenge, but it's one worth the effort to overcome. Even more important is your ability to share information about your situation. Each time you interact with a healthcare provider, you may be expected to provide an accurate medical history, up-to-date medication list, or a brief, detailed description of complaints and symptoms. Having a written history can save you from writing this information repeatedly, especially when you don't feel up to the task. In the future, the Healthcare Information Technology programs will ease this burden by making information available to professionals electronically (see Appendix D).

Doctors seldom look at a patient and make a diagnosis. Assessment begins with history of symptoms and complaints. Labs and image testing won't reveal what a simple complaint of stomach pain before eating can. It is your responsibility to be clear and specific about your signs and symptoms, helping your healthcare provider diagnose and treat you. Preparation and participation will help you obtain the best healthcare possible.

CHAPTER 2

Patient Rights

You may be surprised to learn that you have specific rights when you are a patient, and these are available to you in writing, most often as a handout from the facility's admissions department or upon request from the charge nurse. Documents vary from institution to institution but usually include the following:

- Considerate, respectful care of not only physical illnesses but also spiritual, psychosocial, and cultural-value beliefs
- Impartial access to medically indicated treatment, regardless of race, gender, national origin, disability, sexual orientation, or sources of payment for care
- Honor of advanced directives concerning treatment or designation of a surrogate to make medical decisions
- Clear knowledge of the physician responsible for coordination of care
- Access to information in understandable terms: the diagnosis, treatment, prognosis, and plans for discharge and follow-up
- Ability to make decisions about care and to refuse any or all treatment to the extent permitted by law, and to be informed about the potential medical consequences of such decisions

- Effective management of pain, as appropriate
- Consideration of privacy in all aspects of care, both direct and indirect, expecting that all aspects of your treatment are confidential except as legally reportable. (Note: Some diseases must be reported to state and federal agencies for tracking purposes, such as influenza, food-borne illnesses, sexually transmitted infections, and other communicable diseases.)
- Review and correction of your medical records
- Examination and explanation, if needed, of hospital billing, regardless of source of payment

Printed documents about patient rights may also offer steps to file a written grievance about infringement of those rights, as well as contact information for each state's department of health.

HIPAA Rights to Private and Secure Medical Records

In 1996, the United States Government enacted HIPAA, which stands for the Health Information Portability and Accountability Act, and includes both the Privacy Rule and the Security Rule.

The HIPAA Privacy Rule describes how your health information can be used or disclosed, and who can access your medical information. For example, your medical information cannot be given to your employer or other entity unless you give written authorization. The facility must provide you with information about how your personal information is shared during your first visit or by mail. You can ask for a copy of this at any time.

The Security Rule ensures that your health information is protected. It states what information is to be protected, and what safeguards must be in place to ensure that it is. For example, facilities must provide education to its employees on security of computerized or printed medical records.

HIPAA also grants you the right to inspect, review, and obtain a copy of your medical and billing records held by health plans and healthcare providers. While you may be charged reasonable costs for copying and mailing records, a provider may not deny you a copy of these records because you have not paid for services received (U.S. Department of Health & Human Services, 2012).

If you believe information in your medical or billing records is incorrect, you may request an amendment to the record, and you must receive a response to your request. If the provider or plan does not agree to your request, you have the right to submit a statement of disagreement that must be added to your record.

Understanding your rights as a patient can help you obtain better medical care and ensure your medical records are correct and held in strict confidence.

CHAPTER 3

Using Your Time Well In Healthcare Settings

Whether we like it or not, medicine has become a busier system than ever before. Healthcare is a service, but it is also a business that requires cost control. As the economy has changed, leaving more people without jobs or benefits, increased numbers of patients are using urgent-care clinics or emergency departments as their primary sources of healthcare. Without insurance, people will wait longer to seek medical care, and need more care when they do. For those who have insurance, elective surgeries and those that are not critical may also be put off due to cost.

Insurance, and the paperwork associated with it, uses a tremendous amount of healthcare providers' time. Each insurance program has its own requirements, and many have reduced contract payment to doctors. Clinics and offices are forced to use a managed-care schedule, requiring their providers to see a certain number of patients each hour. For the patient, this results in more time in the waiting room, but a shorter visit with the doctor. The time crunch also affects hospitals, and nurses have increased numbers of patients for which they are responsible. Patients might wait longer after pushing the call button, and receive less individual attention. Overworked staff may be more prone to medication errors. These realities can have a direct impact on your care.

Be Organized

Be organized when you go to an office or clinic visit. Have your specific complaint written down, as well as symptoms, duration, previous attempts at treatment, and the list of all your current medications and supplements. Avoid "doorknob symptoms," those issues patients mention when the doctor's hand is on the doorknob at the end of the appointment. Taking less time to get to the heart of your visit leaves more time for examination and discussion of treatment options.

Symptom logs for new conditions may also help make difficult conditions easier to diagnose. When do you feel light-headed, dizzy, weak, or out of breath? Record date, time, symptom, duration, severity, co-symptoms, and what you were doing at the onset of your symptoms. Make sure you share this with your doctor at your appointment—it will help illuminate patterns that might aid in a diagnosis.

See a Nurse Practitioner or Physician Assistant

Another way to save time is to make appointments for less severe issues with a nurse practitioner or physician assistant. Physicians have treated patients for generations, but as the world of medicine has changed, so has the population of licensed caregivers available to patients. Nurse practitioners (NPs) and physician assistants (PAs) act as "physician extenders," and many patients report that a non-physician caregiver spends more time listening to their complaints, has the same ability to do basic procedures and to write prescriptions as the supervising doctor, and has greater scheduling flexibility.

Differences between Physicians, Physician Assistants, and Nurse Practitioners

While PAs and NPs diagnose and offer treatment, there are slight differences in their function, but not what a typical patient would notice.

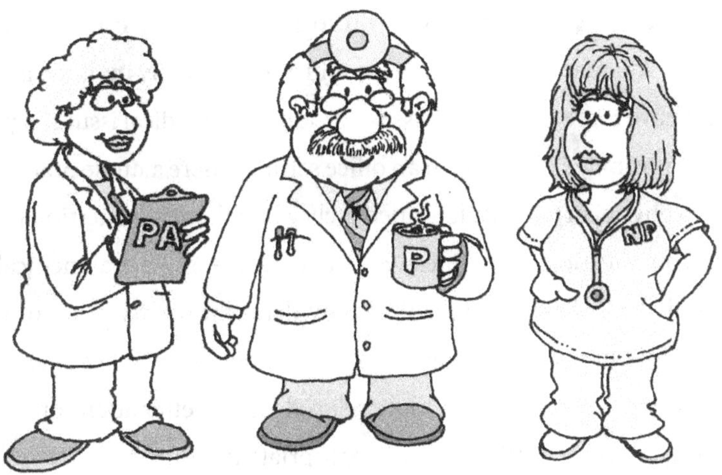

Physicians and Physician Care Extenders

Nurse Practitioner

A nurse practitioner is first a registered nurse who has gone on to receive a master's degree, with additional clinical experience relating to diagnosis and treatment. Specialty areas include acute care, adult health, emergency medicine, family practice, neonatal care, occupational health, oncology, pediatrics, psychiatric and mental health, public health, and women's health. An NP can write prescriptions, order diagnostic tests, and may have hospital privileges. NPs may practice independently in most states.

Physician Assistant

A PA also diagnoses, performs treatment, and writes prescriptions. However, everything a PA does is under the supervision of a licensed physician. Specialty areas include general and internal medicine, orthopedics, geriatrics, family medicine, pediatrics, emergency medicine, general surgery, and thoracic surgery.

What is the advantage for you to see a provider other than your doctor? You may get an appointment in a more-timely manner, and you might have more time to discuss your individual medical issues. A potential disadvantage would be in an office setting where a nurse practitioner has no physician to consult immediately when there is a question regarding a complication of an illness. Still, in rural areas, general medical care certainly beats having no medical providers within fifty miles or more, which does happen. Patients who have had appointments with a physician extender report longer, more relaxed visits, better attention to their medical concerns, and receipt of appropriate treatment.

Have an Advocate

Bringing an advocate is another way to make a visit more efficient. For the same reason that a parent accompanies a child for care, an advocate at an appointment offers an extra set of ears to understand treatments and prognoses, an objective party to ask about something a patient might have forgotten or been reluctant to divulge, and acts as a supportive companion.

Some patients may only need an advocate when facing serious medical issues; others may need someone to assist them with less-acute medical problems, especially when new drugs or diseases are discussed. Making sure the patient understands a new diagnosis and treatment plan is essential. A family member who refuses to take his medication because he "doesn't need it all the time" is one who needs gentle reinforcement about his illness and therapy.

While less an issue when a young adult goes in for a sprained wrist than when an elderly person goes in for shortness of breath, having an advocate who knows a bit about medicine can be invaluable. Finding that someone is not always easy. Ask around. In a pinch, when seeing a physician for an office visit, see if the nurse can be there to answer any questions for you.

When the visit is about test results that could have significant impact on a patient, an advocate is absolutely necessary, even if that person does not have a medical background. No patient hears what a doctor says after the word "cancer," whether it is an actual diagnosis or only a possibility. Some doctors don't seem to consider how devastating such news is, not realizing that further explanation is just noise to the patient trying to wrap his or her head around the disease and its consequences.

Insist that Your Provider Communicate with You

Your provider should speak slowly, clearly, and your language when possible. Don't get lost in medical jargon you don't understand. It's your right to have information in plain language instead of medical terms.

Get Written Instructions

Written instructions are often available for the asking from providers if you're confused about your care or treatment or just want more details about a condition or medication. Read and understand any new prescriptions. If sent electronically, ask your provider to give you a copy of your prescriptions so you can compare when you get to the pharmacy. Pharmacies also offer extensive information about prescribed drugs, so read this before you take the first dose.

Monitor Your Vital Signs

Measure your own vital signs as directed by your healthcare provider. This might only be a monthly blood pressure and pulse check if you're healthy, but may be include a daily weight for patients with congestive heart failure, or blood glucose readings several times a day for those with diabetes. Many monitoring devices, such as blood pressure cuffs, scales, and thermometers, are not expensive. Some insurance companies will even provide such devices at no cost when a patient needs them. Knowing that your medication is working correctly is important to staying healthy. Uncontrolled blood pressure may contribute to heart attack or stroke, but simple home measurement of one's own blood pressure takes about two minutes, is painless, and the recorded results can help healthcare providers plan care.

Blood glucose testing requires a small sample of blood and may be recommended multiple times a day for diabetes that is not well controlled. However, patients may feel that strips are expensive, or that the process is painful and time consuming, so they do not test as directed. Uncontrolled diabetes may lead to complications like kidney failure and blindness. If you have diabetes, follow your healthcare provider's directions for monitoring your disease.

CHAPTER 4

Medical History

Every patient should have a written summary of his or her medical history. Medical history lists more than a patient's diseases and conditions. It should include:

- Current diseases or conditions,
- Previous serious medical problems and surgeries,
- Allergies to medications and other substances,
- Vaccinations,
- Medications and treatments in use (and those previously unsuccessfully attempted), and
- Contact information for all healthcare providers and their specialties.

Your medical history can be written or typed. I strongly suggest that you carry it in a purse or wallet, at least in a condensed form. A small data storage device, such as a thumb drive or micro-SIM in a USB drive adapter provides ease in changing information. Having this information available in a written format can save the effort of having to recall an entire health history each time it is requested, and I recommend this even though future electronic records will be available to healthcare workers.

A Tip for Managing Medical History

It's reasonable to expect to provide your entire medical history to a provider you will see for more than one visit, or for emergency care for an ongoing condition. However, for a minor urgent-care visit in a distant location where treatment is not likely to ever be repeated, it's not necessary to list irrelevant history. A patient with bronchitis or flu while on vacation won't need to recall the broken leg he suffered at age four—but he should definitely share his history of asthma.

SECTION II

WHEN YOU ARE ILL

CHAPTER 5

Disease Management

Knowing What You Have and How it Progresses

There are thousands of diseases. Some are inherited, like hemophilia or Huntington's. Others are caused by a bacteria, virus, or fungus, such as colds, influenza, or athlete's foot. Some have dozens of causes and contributing factors (e.g., emphysema), while others, like cancer, may be caused by outside exposures.

Healthcare providers are familiar with common diseases and conditions, but if you have an unusual disease or condition, you may actually know more about it than your family physician. It is imperative that you and your advocate understand the basics of each disease you have, including the possible complications and how one disease or medication might affect or interfere with one another. A patient who starts Coumadin (warfarin) for an irregular heart rhythm may develop serious bleeding of a stomach ulcer that had not been diagnosed before.

A family practitioner or internal medicine doctor may send you to a specialist, who isn't always aware of your other diagnoses or treatments unless you tell him. Often it's the patient's responsibility to keep all physicians informed, yet the time during an office visit to do so is getting even shorter. A written summary will help ensure that all of your care providers have the same information about your health.

A patient with emphysema may not be able to take certain blood pressure medications due to an interaction between some medications used for each condition. While that information is not commonly recognized by patients, this is a clear example of why patients need to have healthcare providers review all prescribed medications, even those prescribed by other providers.

CHAPTER 6

Treatment Options, Insurance Coverage, and Patients' Rights

Healthcare providers may offer patients the choice of several different treatments. Selecting one, then seeing if it is covered by your insurance, is not for the weak or timid. Dealing with an insurance company can be frustrating and confusing, to say the least. When your insurance company refuses to pay for a procedure it deems "unnecessary" or "experimental," even when your doctor states it is essential, what can you do?

It's not surprising that when insurance companies are trying to curb costs, they limit the treatments they will cover. Many of us saw the movie *John Q* about a father who refused to let the insurance company's policies push his son further from a life-saving heart transplant. While the cost of one heart transplant could pay for hundreds of minor procedures, what is the cost of a little boy's life? And who should be responsible for making such a decision? What if the patient is underinsured or has no insurance?

Often, these financial decisions are viewed as rules, policies, and numbers, not as a suffering patient who needs a life-saving procedure. If a prescribed treatment is not covered, you may need to argue for the care in a civilized manner, and this may require superhuman persistence. Your physician, or someone in her office, may be able to assist in the appeal process if the treatment truly is the best alternative for your care. Exhaust all options before giving up and taking no for a final answer.

Standard of care is a term that applies to all levels of medicine, meaning that the minimum appropriate evidence-based treatment is provided. It's a good phrase to use when discussing disallowed medical care, because in a court of law, judges and juries look for the standard of care to be met. Not all medical care is standard, however. New procedures or medications may not yet be approved by insurance companies. Fortunately, not all necessary care is cutting-edge; occasionally, time-trusted methods are still the best. While pushing for the latest technique isn't always in your best interest, it is also not necessary to accept ineffective treatment if a newer protocol is available.

In the case of a patient who has felt fluttering in her chest on and off for years, but recently has begun to feel light-headed, one cardiologist might recommend treatment with a newer drug. If this medication doesn't work, the physician may decide that ablation (individually identifying and terminating the heart cells that beat out of rhythm) is the next step. This is an invasive and risky procedure. However, another cardiologist might prescribe an older drug with a much longer history of use, finding that it works without any invasive or dangerous interventions. Which protocol is most suitable for this patient? Is cost the most important consideration? Arming yourself with information about your options gives you the best chance at receiving the optimal treatment for your condition.

When considering treatments for organs you cannot replace and cannot live well without, it is reasonable to explore all the possibilities of non-invasive care before stepping into a treatment involving greater risks.

You have only two eyes, for example, and that's one reason why cataract surgery is done one eye at a time—to avoid the risk that some unforeseen, catastrophic problem, such as an infection, might affect both eyes at the same time. You only have one heart, so it makes great sense to have a second opinion before non-emergent diagnostic tests or procedures, like a cardiac catheterization or pacemaker implantation. Be leery of the physician who is not willing to arrange for your receipt of a second opinion.

Your most important right as a patient when you are not comfortable with the direction of your care is the right to refuse. When you feel that your physician is not offering a reasonable list of options, isn't listening

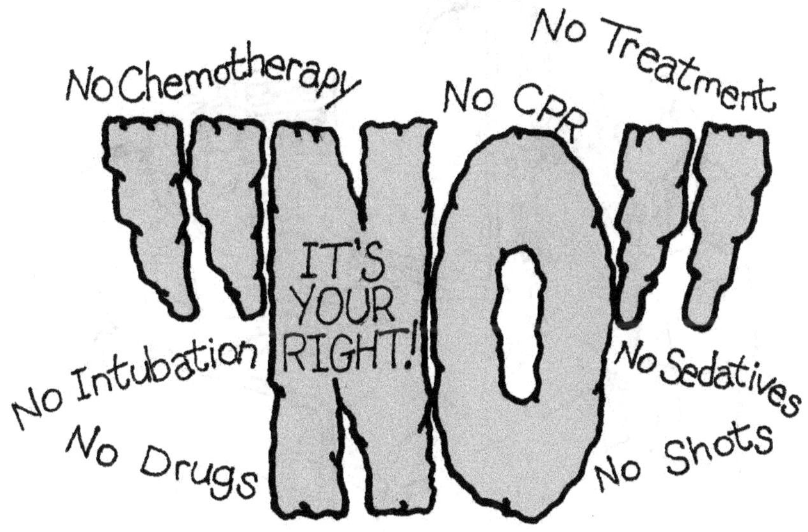

It's your right to just say no.

to you as a patient, or perhaps is not concerned about the side effects or complications that worry you, it is your right to refuse care.

Refusing a treatment or procedure and standing up for yourself against a healthcare provider might feel uncomfortable, but it could also open communication toward finding a better alternative for your care. You may exercise this right of refusal anytime a healthcare provider directs treatment or diagnostic testing, regardless of whether you are an inpatient or an outpatient.

My mother's cardiologist once prescribed a different class of blood-pressure medication than she had been using. The directions were to take one tablet a day for two weeks, then to take two tablets a day. After several days of taking only one tablet, her blood pressure was so low she was unable to get up and safely walk to the bathroom. At my insistence, she called the doctor to advise him of what was happening to her. Through his nurse, the doctor stated that he expected her to "follow his directions

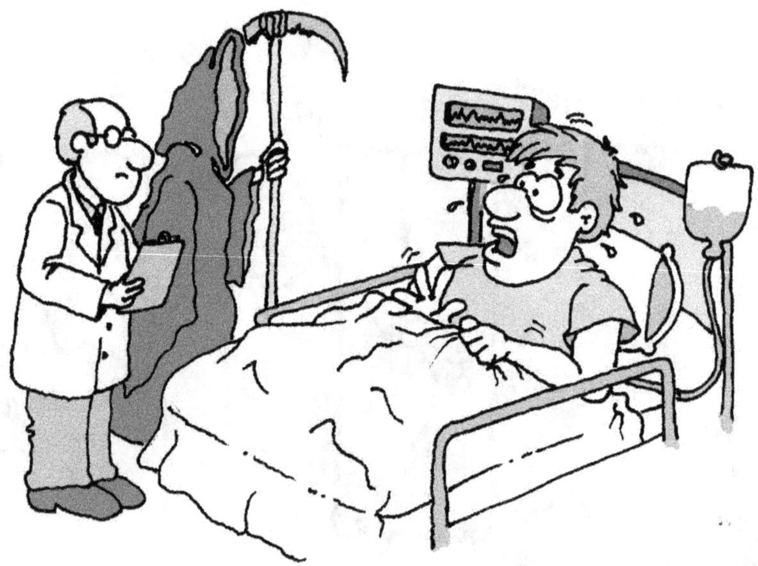

Complications to your surgery include death...

or else." Advocating for her, I suggested she take the "or else" option, since she was not tolerating the drug and her health was worsening because of it. My advocacy helped her understand the medical issue and her right to refuse the doctor's treatment option, so that she could protect her health.

You have rights as a patient, but it is up to you to exercise them. You have the right to understand all protocols of care, to have these presented in language you understand, and to investigate options. The informed consent you provide, in writing, before undergoing surgery lists what could go wrong. You also have the right to ask the physician to explain every action or task involved in the surgery, if you desire. A surgeon who will not take the time to answer your questions might not be the one you want elbow-deep in your intestines, right?

While any medical procedure carries risks, such as uncontrolled bleeding or even death, you have the right to understand the likelihood of these events occurring and to weigh them against the potential benefits of the procedure for improving your health. If the benefits do not sufficiently outweigh the risks to you, you have the right to refuse the procedure.

Another right you have as a patient is the right to correctly billed medical care. Surprisingly, insurance companies may not take the time to evaluate a bill before paying it so long as nothing unusual appears. Sometimes, even really outrageous charges get ignored, as happened in the case of a breast reduction. The hospital billed—and was paid for—a pair of breast *implants*.

Obtain and review itemized bills for all of your procedures and hospitalizations. Overbilling is an unfortunate and commonly accepted mistake in American medicine. If your insurance company will not work to reconcile overcharges, you still should. If you believe that your billing was intentionally fraudulent, contact your insurance representative so it may be investigated.

CHAPTER 7

Having Someone to Advocate for Your Care

Obtaining a patient advocate is the most valuable step you can take to make healthcare more effective, particularly when dealing with a serious condition or disease. Adults take children to the doctor, listen to the diagnosis, ask questions, and discuss treatments. That's advocacy. At some point, a patient is old enough to obtain medical care for himself, and is seldom in need of an advocate. When the diagnosis is a sprained wrist or a simple laceration, having an advocate isn't critical.

> **ad•vo•cate** – *noun* In the medical field, a person who focuses on bolstering the patient's role and rights in making decisions about his or her healthcare.
> *http://medical-dictionary.thefreedictionary.com/advocate*

Imagine being in the hospital for abdominal pain that has not gone away despite multiple trials of medication. When the doctor comes to the bedside and announces that you have colon cancer, nothing else he says makes any sense. The diagnosis is so shocking, it ends all rational interpretation for you, the patient. This kind of news can come in most any situation, from a normal pregnancy with an unexplained death of the baby just before delivery, to a previously healthy woman with a hip fracture who develops a blood clot in her leg during her recovery. When we need someone to help us listen, understand, and

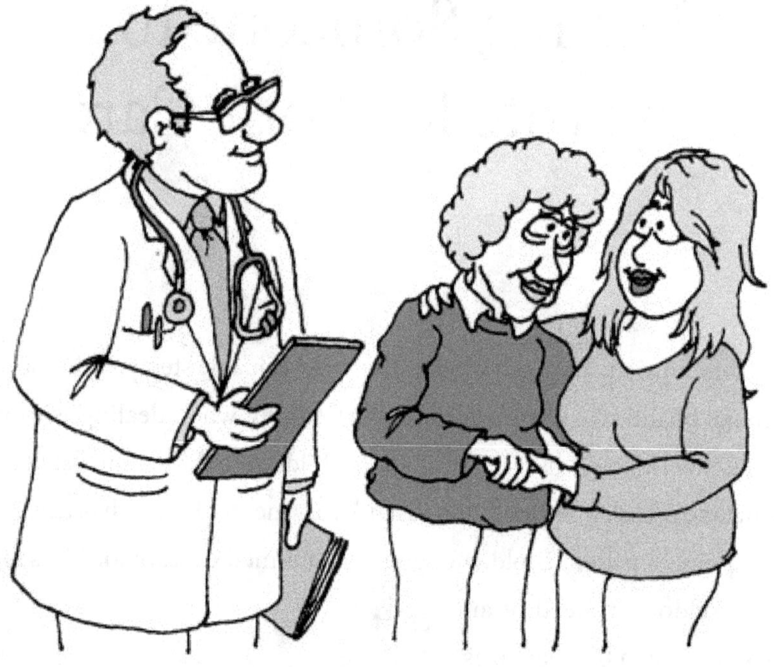

ask questions, an advocate provides that valuable assistance.

In many cases, a family member can adequately advocate for a patient, but there are times when diagnoses or treatment options will overwhelm everyone in the family. In today's world, having a friend or other trusted person who can be an effective advocate is important, though perhaps harder to accomplish. Finding an advocate who understands your wishes and can remain objective, focus on the diagnosis, and help you plan for the next steps for treatment can help you do better in the long run, simply because someone is available assist with getting more complete answers and to discuss options.

Advocacy is not decision by committee; it doesn't take a dozen people to hear a problem and determine a solution. A room full of siblings discussing a parent's care often ends in confusion as options turn into arguments. Whenever possible, the patient needs to make his own decisions, with the assistance of an emotionally objective advocate. It is not the responsibility of the patient to make everyone happy.

I knew a patient who was a 90-year-old woman with Alzheimer's dementia. She was diagnosed with cancer of the liver, pancreas, and lymph nodes. Against the patient's written wishes from several years prior, when she was of sound mental capacity, her family wanted her to have radiation therapy for six weeks. Doctors told the family that the radiation would not cure her cancer, and she had no significant pain at this time, so treatment was not even for pain control. Because this patient could no longer speak for herself, emotionally charged family members disregarded her wishes and directed her healthcare, in this case subjecting her to a four-hour round-trip drive, five days a week, to obtain the radiation therapy.

No one lives forever, and as hard as it is to make a decision that treatment is worse than the disease, there comes a time when family must make the right decision for the patient.

For situations when a patient cannot make or state a decision for himself, the importance of documents like a Living Will, Advanced Directive, or Durable Power of Attorney for Healthcare can help delineate the decision tree, and in many cases will clarify the patient's decision made before the situation becomes critical.

CHAPTER 8

Tips About Health Conditions From Other Patients

Because healthcare providers don't suffer all the diseases they treat, other patients may be the best source of information on how to actually live with conditions. The quality of that advice will, of course, need to be evaluated. In many cases, support groups or organizations for specific diseases or conditions are available to provide critical information, offer self-help hints, and provide avenues for connection with others who are living with the condition. From autoimmune diseases to traumatic injuries, there are websites and other social networking resources for patients or their families to explore. Often, realizing you are not alone in facing your condition can be a good first step toward learning how to live with it.

Below are some common conditions and a few tips, such as you might learn from a support group. In some cases, lifestyle choices can be powerful in improving health, even though the disease itself cannot be cured.

Emphysema

There is no cure for emphysema, however, early recognition and treatment can help slow the progression of the disease. So symptoms and treatment recommendations should be heeded. One major piece of advice, which is often ignored, is to stop smoking. I've heard patients say there's no reason to quit after being diagnosed, but that's not true. Quitting, as difficult as it can be, will help improve the efficiency of the lungs, making each breath work better. It's not a cure, but quitting smoking does help slow the progression of lung damage.

Because emphysema inhibits a patient's capacity to breathe efficiently, use of a ventilator was once the only option for assisting respirations when seriously ill. No one wants to be intubated and on a ventilator, but keeping the body well oxygenated and letting the patient rest from the exhausting effort of breathing may be worth the inconvenience. More recently, non-invasive breathing-assist machines are used in hospitals, allowing patients in respiratory distress a new option. Use of such ventilation assistance like CPAP (used by many at home for sleep apnea) and BiPAP allows a patient ease in breathing, resting heart and skeletal muscles, and reducing the demand on the lungs to provide oxygen for the body.

Heart Disease

Cardiovascular diseases include enlargement of the heart, impaired cardiac-muscle function from damage, or chronic rhythm disturbance. Because the diseased heart is less able to perform at its peak, other organ systems begin to suffer the effects of poor circulation. These may include swelling to the legs, fluid in the lungs, or blood clots. It's important to follow your doctor's advice for medications; it's equally important to understand what those prescribed medications do and how they should be helping. Medications prescribed to remove excess fluid, which the body may store as swelling in the feet, legs, or lungs, often are accompanied by strict weight-measurement instructions. Water weighs about seven pounds per gallon, so a weight gain of more than three or four pounds can indicate swelling of half a gallon in body tissues. This swelling is easily monitored with daily weight checks.

> For more ideas on diet, visit the Mayo Clinic website at:
>
> *http://www.mayoclinic.com/health/cholesterol/CL00002*

Patients with heart disease might have dietary restrictions Salt will cause retention of water, so a low-sodium diet is often recommended. Canned foods have particularly high amounts of salt. Choosing from a low-cholesterol menu is also helpful: more fresh vegetables and fruits; oatmeal and high-fiber foods; omega-3 meats such as salmon, mackerel, halibut, and albacore tuna; nuts; and small amounts of olive oil for sautéing vegetables, dipping bread, or basting meat are all excellent choices.

If allowed, an exercise program can help condition muscles, including the heart, making their use of available oxygen and nutrients more efficient. Again, smoking wastes lung capacity that is better used for changing body needs. The goal is to make more oxygen available, and to make organs better able to use it.

Many cardiac patients take Coumadin (a brand name for warfarin). Coumadin does not actually "thin" the blood, but increases the time needed for blood to form a clot by inhibiting an enzyme that interferes with Vitamin K metabolism. In patients with atrial fibrillation or atrial flutter, the top two chambers of the heart do not contract in an organized manner, which may allow blood to stagnate in the chamber edges where it can form clots. Depending on the location in the heart, these clots can move into circulation, affecting the heart itself, lungs, brain, or extremities. Other patients may have blood clots in the veins of their legs, which can break loose and circulate to the lungs. Coumadin helps prevent these clots from forming.

Because drugs like Coumadin alter clotting of blood, healthcare providers monitor blood coagulation times by a lab test on a small sample. However, Coumadin and similar drugs can cause minor bleeding, such as bruising, or serious, life-threatening bleeding such as massive internal hemorrhage. Due to this effect, monitoring is mandatory for all patients taking Coumadin. Patients who take other coagulation-altering medications should be monitored until the response is determined to be within range. Some patients who take Coumadin become stable on a regular dose. Others have lab values that vary significantly so the dose requires frequent adjustment. Another oddity is the dose required for Coumadin to meet therapeutic goals because it can vary widely from one patient to another. Dosage for appropriate anti-coagulation may range from 1 mg to 10 mg per day.

Cancer

There are hundreds of types of cancers, each with its own prognosis and treatment protocol. Some cancers spread to other organs quickly, while others remain contained. It's important that a patient understand the implications and options of his specific cancer diagnosis. One very helpful website is produced by the American Cancer Society, and has many pages on types of cancer and treatment therapies at *http://www.*

cancer.org. Another good resource is *http://www.cancer.gov/*.

One type of treatment is chemotherapy, which includes the use of a single drug or combination of drugs that will target cancer cells. While the cancer is the target, chemotherapy affects the whole body. Appetite is one of the areas caught in the crossfire between treatment and result—food simply does not taste the same. A bite of lemon or lime can help to reset the taste buds for a meal, and the citrus aroma might also help reduce the nausea associated with chemo. Ginger also reduces nausea when used with foods. Choosing a pleasant lotion and lip balm may counter the drying effects of the chemotherapy.

Another type of treatment is radiation therapy. Because it is more focused, radiation treatment can cause skin burns. It is also exhausting, and rest is critical to healing. Even an hour's nap each day can be helpful in boosting energy and keeping a patient active.

Some types of cancer can cause severe, chronic pain that is untouched by less-than-massive doses of narcotic pain medications. One complaint I hear from cancer and other chronic pain patients is how others do not acknowledge their level of pain. It's not a visible symptom. Often the patient just muddles through the day, so family and friends cannot understand the full impact pain has. Chronic pain leaves a patient exhausted but feeling she must just keep going, or lie down and give up. It's important for loved ones to remember, even though you don't see cancer, it can be excruciatingly painful.

Cancer and other debilitating diseases may leave a patient homebound. While visitors are usually welcome, sometimes a patient just cannot muster the energy to be a good host or hostess. Family and friends should not be offended if a patient does not feel up to seeing them at a certain time. In a hospital setting, patients and advocates might ask the nursing staff to intervene, restricting visitation or limiting the time visitors can stay.

At home, a sign for the patient's front door might be helpful: it may read "Please come in to visit," or "I'm not up for your visit today." A notepad and pen so visitors could leave a note saying they'd dropped by might also work well.

Another helpful tip is to have a chore book. Many times, visitors want to know what they can do, but the patient or family may hesitate to ask too much. A chore book lists daily, weekly, or occasional tasks that need doing: washing the dishes, watering the houseplants, mowing the lawn, or picking up milk and bread. A list gives those who wish to do something a choice of tasks, and they simply pencil in the date they did the chore, so the next person knows when it was done last.

One other thing homebound patients or their advocates can ask of those who offer is a prepared meal—something that takes little effort to fix, might be a favorite of the patient, or can be frozen for later use. Caring for a loved one at home takes all the energy some caregivers have, leaving little for preparing healthy meals for themselves or the patient.

Autoimmune Diseases

Autoimmune conditions encompass more than 80 diseases affecting 23.5 million people. Most autoimmune diseases, such as multiple sclerosis, myasthenia gravis, lupus, and rheumatoid arthritis, have no cure. Many have no visible symptoms, can be difficult to measure or assess in their early stages. Patients often go through elimination of dozens of other medical conditions first, and doctors may dismiss complaints because lab tests and other measures come back as negative. Worse, friends and family, who can't see many of the symptoms, may be unsympathetic to the real limitations a patient faces every day.

Multiple sclerosis affects the ability of the brain and spinal cord to communicate when the nerves lose the protective sheath called myelin. This can cause almost any neurological symptom: pain, loss of sensation, or physical and cognitive disruption. Patients with multiple sclerosis often search out treatments or lifestyle changes that help with their symptoms when traditional medical therapy fails to help. Dietary choices, vitamin and herbal supplements, alternative medicine therapies, such as acupuncture, and stress reduction are options that may offer relief. A helpful website to begin researching autoimmune diseases is *http://www.aarda.org/*.

Alzheimer's and Other Dementia Conditions

There are a number of disease processes that rob a person of his or her mental function, including Alzheimer's and senile dementia. To attempt to write about them and their effects on loved ones in such a short description is impossible, but I would like to share a website devoted to patients and families: *www.alz.org*. This site is dedicated to offering information about the signs and symptoms of Alzheimer's, explanations about its progression, updates on research, and a 24-hour hotline.

Patients with early dementia often realize something is wrong, which may cause embarrassment and increase their reluctance to seek medical assistance. At some point, there is no hiding the symptoms from those around them, however, which may be frustrating to an independent person. If you can imagine how exasperating it is to misplace your car in a parking lot, imagine the enormity of being unable to remember where your house is.

Alzheimer's patients often progress toward one of two extremes—they may become pleasant and polite in their diminished memories, easily redirected to an alternate task, or they may become aggressive toward those around them, sometimes even physically violent. In either case, loved ones may struggle to cope with the "loss" of their family member's ability to remember them. I offer this guidance: the patient can't change how he thinks now, and there is no point in arguing with or correcting him in the later stages of dementia. Enjoy the lucid moments, but don't expect them. Being frustrated will only create upset in a patient who doesn't know what is being asked, and thus cannot respond appropriately.

In many dementia patients' lives, there comes a point where independent living is no longer possible. As much as families don't want to consider nursing facilities, living with or caring for the patient full-time may become unfeasible. In later stages, placement in a secure Alzheimer's facility may be the most caring measure that can be taken, providing a safe, monitored environment focused on the needs of patients with dementia.

Another consideration is the patient's wishes for life-extending treatments. The family may be asked to make do-not-resuscitate decisions, and may need to acknowledge that a dementia patient who survives a cardiac arrest will not come back in better condition.

As I noted before, the list of diseases and the resources for them is extensive, but it is important to begin gathering information from credible sources. For further information about these and other diseases and conditions, the Centers for Disease Control and Prevention website, features a searchable list—*http://www.cdc.gov/DiseasesConditions.*

CHAPTER 9

Emergency Preparedness

Disasters such as tornadoes, hurricanes or earthquakes can have catastrophic effects on an individual's medical care. Being prepared for an emergency means planning for a catastrophic event affecting hundreds or thousands of people, or a facing a disaster as limited as a house fire or death in the family requiring immediate travel.

If you take medication regularly, emergency preparedness includes the following:

- Store copies of your prescription labels somewhere besides where your drugs are kept. Replacement, if it becomes necessary, will be easier when the pharmacy number, location, prescription number, and other data are at your fingertips.
- Keep at least three days' worth of medications available, separate from the main bottles. Remember, also, that it's illegal to carry unmarked medications. Ask your pharmacy for extra bottles with labels. Place each medication in its own bottle—don't mix them.
- Maintain a current medical history and medication list.
- If you use oxygen, be prepared for weather-related interruptions,

such as power outages or delivery delays due to snowstorms. You may need permission from your insurance company, but in many cases when a weather event is predicted, oxygen suppliers may make an exception to keep you supplied.

Other tips for emergency preparedness include:

- Know when to evacuate. Get out of situations where your health may be at risk before there is a crisis. For example, consider evacuating your home early when there are wildfires in the area, especially if you need someone to assist you. Leave before smoke affects your respiratory ailment, impairing your ability to function.
- Have a plan with family members. Know where to meet after an emergency such as a house fire or tornado. Knowing where to find and be found by others will reduce the panic of the situation.
- Put together a survival kit. This should include at least three days' worth of food, water, medicine and other essentials, along with flashlights, a battery-powered radio, and a whistle. Depending on where you live, this kit may be best kept in your tornado shelter or other location.
- Know the location of your evacuation center and whether it will take a pet if you need to take one, or if you have severe allergies to animals that might be present.
- If you have diabetes and end up in an evacuation center, you will need to know how to store your insulin, and about switching insulin types in an emergency if a refill is not immediately available.
- Plan for winter-weather emergencies, both beforehand and

during a storm. Make your home as weatherproof as possible. Have a safe alternate heating source if the main system is electric, but make sure that any combustible heat source is vented properly, and that smoke detectors and carbon monoxide detectors are working. Have a week's worth of water and food that does not require cooking or refrigeration, such as canned or dried food (and keep a non-electric can opener handy).

- Flooding can potentially affect large areas for a long time, making evacuation necessary, sanitation a huge problem, and re-entering a residence dangerous. Standing or wading in water cooler than 75 degrees can lead to hypothermia as body heat is washed away.
- Extreme summer heat can be an emergency in parts of the country when temperatures and humidity soar, leaving the power grid to struggle as air conditioners and fans try to keep up. The elderly, the very young, and those with chronic medical problems are especially at risk because of their poor body temperature regulation and their reduced ability to escape their homes to cooler locales. Heat-related illnesses and deaths are preventable, yet they still occur. Never leave anyone in a vehicle, no matter how brief an errand might be. The temperature in a parked car can become incapacitating and fatal in just minutes.
- A cellular phone, even a pay-as-you-go or limited-access-use unit, can make travel safer and offer portable communication in an emergency. Even a phone without a paid service is able to contact 911.
- For those who live alone, or who are alone during portions of the day, a button-emergency system can be a lifesaver in the event of a fall or other medical crisis.

In major disasters, being self-reliant for the first three days is the key to survival. Looking back at Hurricane Katrina, lives were lost when residents did not evacuate. As has happened before in other disasters, many of those who stayed did not have a plan to be self-sustaining for the time it took rescuers to reach them. Unfortunately, not all emergencies come with the same warning to prepare, so it is up to you to be ready for whatever disaster might affect you.

> The United States Government offers useful emergency planning information online:
>
> *http://www.ready.gov/*
> *http://www.fema.gov/plan/index.shtm*
> *http://www.bt.cdc.gov/*

CHAPTER 10

Vaccinations for Viral Diseases

One way to stay healthier is to stay up to date on recommended vaccines. Immunizations for such viruses as seasonal influenza and pneumonia can be lifesaving protection, especially for those with existing health concerns. Those who have frequent contact with family and close friends with compromised health should also be immunized to reduce the risk of passing on preventable communicable infections. For example, if a woman with emphysema lives with her daughter and son-in-law, all three should receive vaccinations for flu and pneumonia. Grandparents who will be around a newborn may need a pertussis vaccination.

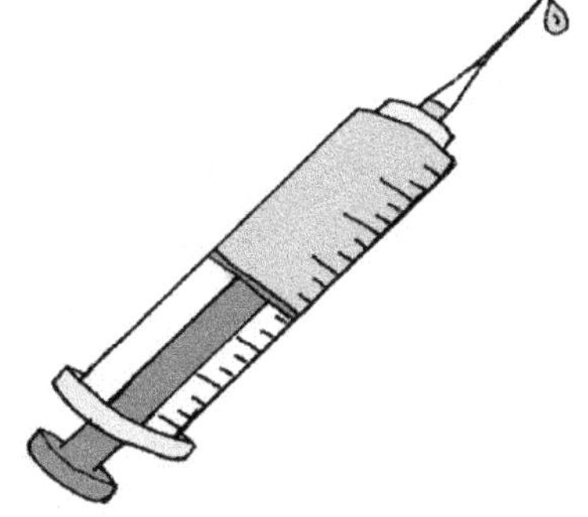

Most adults need not be concerned about catching pertussis (whooping cough). Some may have had it without ever having been diagnosed, suffering the long-lasting cough and other respiratory symptoms with only moderate distress. However, infants and small children are seriously affected by the exhausting relentless cough, some suffering life-threatening breathing impairment. Most cases of infant pertussis in recent years have been traced to an adult family member or close friend who has not been properly vaccinated. Infants under six months of age are not yet protected by pertussis vaccine, so anyone who is going to be around a newborn should be immunized for pertussis.

Adult Vaccinations

Tetanus: Tetanus or "lockjaw" causes painful tightening of the muscles, usually all over the body. It can lead to "locking" of the jaw so the victim cannot open his mouth or swallow. Tetanus leads to death in about 1 in 10 cases. Typically combined with diphtheria (TD), most people need this vaccine every 10 years. Tetanus, diphtheria and pertussis (TDaP) can be given at any time if needed, even if the 10 years has not passed since the last TD dose.

MMR (measles, mumps, rubella): These "childhood diseases" of past generations have been controlled with immunizations in recent generations. Update at 19 to 49 years of age, one or two doses; over 50, one more dose if at risk.

Chickenpox: Varicella or chickenpox is a highly contagious disease that is very uncomfortable and sometimes serious. If a patient has not had his disease, the vaccination is two doses.

Zoster (shingles): Shingles is a painful localized skin rash, often with blisters, that is caused by the varicella zoster virus (VZV), the same virus that causes chickenpox. Anyone who has had chickenpox can develop shingles because VZV remains in the nerve cells of the body. One dose is recommended for those over 60 years of age.

Hepatitis A: A serious liver disease caused by a virus that is spread by the fecal-oral route, where an object or food contaminated with the stool of a person with hepatitis A is put into another person's mouth. Two doses.

Hepatitis B: Hepatitis B is a serious disease caused by a virus that can cause lifelong infection, cirrhosis (scarring) of the liver, liver cancer, liver failure, and death. It is spread through exposure to contaminated bodily fluids. Three doses.

Meningitis: Infection of the covering of the brain and spinal cord; can be either caused by a virus or bacteria. One or two doses for those at risk. Many universities are now mandating this immunization as a requirement for general admission in certain age groups, especially if living in dorms, and specifically for programs in healthcare and education. Investigate requirements ahead of time as there are often shortages of this and other vaccinations.

HPV (human papillomavirus): HPV vaccines protect against human papillomavirus (HPV) infection and HPV-related disease. Three doses in late pre-teen and teenage girls and boys are now recommended. Some advertising claimed that this vaccine prevents some types of gynecological cancer. This is not exactly true—the vaccine prevents infections that have been linked to these cancers, but it does not prevent the cancer directly. It also does not protect from all types of HPV virus.

Pneumonia: Caused by *Streptococcus pneumoniae* infection of the lungs, the most common disease caused by this bacterium in adults. For patients 19 to 64 years of age, one or two shots may be given if the patient is at risk. After age 65, only one dose is necessary, even if previous vaccination had been received.

Influenza: Influenza A causes moderate-to-severe illness, and affects all age groups. Influenza B generally causes milder disease than type A, and primarily affects children. This vaccination is offered annually in the fall and needs to be received every year to be effective. Manufacturers create a vaccine each year, targeting the most probable strains of influenza. As with many of the vaccines, immunization does not guarantee you will not get the disease, but the vaccination offers increased protection from those specific strains. If you do get sick, you will often have a less-severe case.

There are dozens of other adult immunizations available. The Centers for Disease Control alters recommendations frequently, but this list is current at the time of this publication. Immunizations are recommended for people at particular risk.

This includes those who may be exposed to diseases (or may expose others) in their home and work environments (e.g., healthcare providers or family members of infants or small children), or those who have chronic diseases.

For those who travel overseas, review necessary vaccinations in advance as some require multiple doses over several months. Some of the immunizations you might need include polio, anthrax, smallpox, Lyme disease, plague, typhoid, and yellow fever. Rabies vaccination is also available for those in high-risk professions, as well as those exposed through an animal bite.

CHAPTER 11

Drug-Resistant Diseases

The discovery of antibiotics is perhaps one of the most important advances in health in human history, decreasing suffering from disease and saving lives. Unfortunately, we've reached a time when overuse and misuse of antibiotics have led to dangerous consequences.

The use and misuse of antimicrobials in human medicine and animal husbandry over the past 70 years has led to a relentless rise in the number and types of microorganisms resistant to these medicines—leading to death, increased suffering and disability, and higher healthcare costs (World Health Organization, 2010a).

The key to success in treating bacterial infections is prompt and correct administration of antibiotics. It has been the inappropriate and indiscriminate use of antibiotics, often for infections that are not of bacterial origin, which has led to drug-resistant microbes. Antibiotics do not have any effect on viral infections.

A bacterial infection the media has brought to light is MRSA (sometimes pronounced as a word, "mer-sa"): methicillin-resistant *Staphylococcus aureus*. Normal treatment with antibiotics, and even with methicillin, no longer controls this bacterium. MRSA is one of a growing number of resistant diseases of varying communicability.

The common form of *Staphylococcus aureus*, the bacteria that causes Staph infections, is an ordinary bacterium for humans, common on our skin and in our environment. The problem is that those who have misused or overused antibiotics carry and spread the infection. This has led to the bacterial infection becoming less curable by standard antibiotics, in this case beta-lactams, including methicillin, thus the name methicillin-resistant.

MRSA is a very hardy bacterium with the ability to survive on surfaces for an extended period of time. In daycare and school settings where children may spread MRSA, prisons and shelters with close quarters, or employees handling food or producing livestock, this bacterium has become both more prolific and more difficult to control. In a hospital setting, any patient with open wounds is at risk of acquiring this infection because it survives on so many surfaces in care areas. Worse still, healthcare providers may be unknown carriers of the bacteria, not having any symptoms but contaminating patients and patient-care areas.

Some facts about bacterial infections:

- Infections caused by resistant microorganisms often fail to respond to conventional treatment, resulting in prolonged illness and greater risk of death. This is especially true in patients who are being treated for other medical conditions.
- A high percentage of hospital-acquired infections are caused by highly resistant bacteria, such as MRSA.
- About 440,000 new cases of multidrug-resistant tuberculosis (MDR-TB) emerge annually, causing at least 150,000 deaths worldwide. In the United States, 11,182 cases of TB were reported in 2010, a slight decrease; however, Hispanics and Asians still

account for over half the cases reported. More than 1% of the total U.S. cases are multi-drug resistant.

For more information on tuberculosis in the U.S., visit the Centers for Disease Control website at:

http://www.cdc.gov/tb/statistics/reports/2010/pdf/report2010.pdf

- Resistance to earlier generation anti-malarial medicines, such as chloroquine and sulfadoxine-pyrimethamine, is now widespread in most malaria-endemic countries, affecting those who travel.
- Inappropriate and irrational use of antimicrobial medicines provides favorable conditions for resistant microorganisms to emerge, spread, and persist (World Health Organization, 2010).

In most cases, most resistant bacterial infections can be treated and cured. Antibiotic treatment of MRSA infections requires intravenous vancomycin, a drug requiring pharmacy-directed dosing because its therapeutic window between effectiveness and toxicity is very narrow. Patients receiving such intravenous infusions will undergo frequent lab testing to assure that they are getting the correct dose.

Unfortunately, even resistance to vancomycin has become an issue with *Staphylococcus* and *Enterococcus* bacterium. Drug resistance and multi-drug resistance is also of increasing concern in tuberculosis, *Pseudomonas, Clostridium, Salmonella, Escherichia coli* (E. coli), *Acinetobacter* and other bacteria in the last five years. *USA Today* reported in September 2010 about a "superbug" that was completely resistant to all drugs: a strain of *Klebsiella pneumoniae* that has been found in 35 states so far and has a fatality rate of 30 to 60%. Recent good news from England, however, shows rates of MRSA and *Clostridium* infection in the U.K. have fallen.

Healthcare Providers Should Their Wash Hands

It's your right to have care provided by staff that washes their hands and uses appropriate protective devices to prevent the spread of disease to you.

You absolutely have the right to ask, or demand if required, that your nurse, technician, doctor, or other provider wash his or her hands before touching you.

How do you take care of yourself against such a powerful list of infectious bacteria?

- Start by staying healthy.
- Wash your hands often.
- Do not touch your eyes or contact lenses without washing your hands first.
- Use, but do not overuse, cleaners and decontamination solutions for home or personal use. For example, use a sanitizing hand gel after looking at a menu or pushing a shopping cart, but not more often than you would wash your hands if you had facilities available.
- Be diligent in settings where contamination is likely to occur, such as doctors' offices, grocery stores, and public transportation. Use alcohol-based cleanser before carrying germs from these areas to your car or into your household.
- Clean commonly touched surfaces in your household, especially when someone is sick. Refrigerator handles, doorknobs, faucets,

stair rails, etc., are all are where places bacteria and viruses can be transferred from one person to another.

- Avoid touching surfaces where contamination is most likely to be found, such as chairs in a doctor's waiting room, or any hospital equipment when visiting. Wash your hands thoroughly before and after.
- Demand that healthcare providers who intend to render care wash their hands in your room and wear appropriate gloves, masks, and gowns when indicated, especially when you have open wounds or are in an already immune-compromised state. Doctors are especially guilty of not doing this as they make rounds from room to room. IT IS YOUR RIGHT.
- Do not ask for antibiotics for every respiratory ailment or other minor infection. Trust your physician to make the right call whether the infection requires an antibiotic. Infections in relatively healthy humans should begin to clear up within a few days. If they don't, revisit the need for antibiotics.
- If prescribed antibiotics, finish them as directed.
- Consider getting annual flu vaccinations. Preventing or controlling a viral infection can lessen the chances it could be complicated by a secondary bacterial infection, such as a simple cold causing a patient to be more susceptible to a sinus infection or pneumonia.

SECTION III

END-OF-LIFE DECISION MAKING

CHAPTER 12

End-of-Life Choices

DNR / Living Will / Advanced Directives / Durable Power of Attorney for Healthcare

Regardless of age, adult patients should consider, discuss with family members, and make written directives about their wishes for treatment if suffering critical injuries, an unexpected outcome occurs, or in the event of a terminal disease.

Three documents are important for you to understand:

1. the DNR (do not resuscitate),
2. Living Will or Advanced Directives, and
3. Durable Power of Attorney for Healthcare.

Knowing the circumstances when each is appropriate is important. Each document is instantly revocable by the patient, which means that you can have one, but can change your mind about it at any time.

It is also essential that you know that in most cases, a Do-Not-Resuscitate order properly executed by the patient can be overridden by the patient's family. For example, a mother of seven adult children has a DNR for a hospital stay when she suffers a cardiac arrest. Six of those children may agree to follow her wishes and the DNR, but if the seventh child tells healthcare staff to "do everything to save her," that one individual's wishes will likely be followed instead of those of the document or other family members. Healthcare workers opt to defend themselves for treating rather than for not treating a patient. A frank discussion of your expectations in the event of an emergency with those who may be asked to decide on your behalf can help ensure your wishes will be honored.

Irreversible or Terminal Conditions

Patients and families must understand that "irreversible conditions" are those illnesses, injuries or conditions that:

1. May be treated but will never be cured,
2. Will leave a patient unable to care for or to make decisions for him/herself, and
3. Without medical life-sustaining treatment in accordance with the standard of care, the condition is fatal.

An "irreversible" condition is not necessarily a "terminal" condition. Consider the horrible case of Terri Schiavo, for whom medical decisions were argued by biological family, her husband, and eventually the legal system. Terri had collapsed in cardiac arrest at home and was subsequently diagnosed by the medical team as being in a persistent vegetative state. The initial arguments were about removing her feeding tube, on which she relied for nutrition and hydration. Her condition of persistent vegetative state was irreversible, but it was not terminal. She was dependent on the use of the tube feedings for her survival, just as you and I are on having our meals, but she was not going to die immediately without them as she would have had she been on a ventilator supporting her breathing.

On the other hand, "terminal" applies to a patient condition, injury or illness that will be the direct cause of death, typically with a prognosis of length of survival. Terminal conditions cannot be reversed, such as some cancers or end-stage failure of an organ system. Terminal patients who are in the last days or hours of life do not have a physiological need for nutrition or hydration. As a body goes through the dying process, gastric function ceases, making tube feedings useless and possibly even uncomfortable; hydration is no longer being absorbed by the cells and may cause swelling of arms and legs. Although a conscious patient should be made comfortable, including intake as desired, restriction of nutrition and hydration in an actively dying unconscious patient should not be considered withholding of necessary care.

Living Will

Many serious illnesses may be described as irreversible early in the course of the illness, but they may not be considered terminal until the disease is fairly advanced, such as with emphysema or kidney disease. In thinking about terminal illness and its treatment, you may wish to consider the relative benefits and burdens of treatment throughout the course of the disease, and discuss your wishes with your physician, family, and important persons in your life. When your healthcare team and family know ahead of time what your wishes are, they can adhere to them.

Each state's documentation differs and should be evaluated specifically. In Texas, for example, a Living Will document includes a Medical

Power of Attorney: Directive to Physicians and Family or Surrogates. A New Mexico Living Will document also includes end-of-life decisions regarding withdrawal or withholding of treatment, including artificial nutrition and hydration. Different states and healthcare providers may interpret continued nutrition and hydration as treatment for a patient who is in a non-responsive state but not for a patient who is truly in the last days or hours of life.

Depending on the document, Advanced Directives may include the wishes that, under certain circumstances of physician evaluation, all treatments except comfort care be withheld, allowing the patient to die, or that all life-sustaining treatments be utilized even in a terminal condition (with the exception of Hospice patients).

Durable Power of Attorney for Healthcare

A Durable Power of Attorney for Healthcare is not the same as a general Power of Attorney. A Power of Attorney gives authorization to make decisions regarding financial and legal matters, whereas a Durable Power of Attorney for Healthcare (DPAH) solely directs medical choices while the patient is cognitively incapacitated or unable to make or state a medical decision for himself. The DPAH is written by the patient and names someone as the decision-maker regarding healthcare for the patient only in the event the patient cannot make decisions or verbalize them for himself. When a woman undergoes a planned appendix removal, she will sign the consents for the surgery herself, but if the doctor finds a cancerous ovarian tumor during the surgery, he may seek permission from the DPAH designee to do a hysterectomy during that surgery rather than take the patient to surgery a second time.

Although I recommend all patients have a DPAH, I also advise caution when a patient chooses to name a Power of Attorney. When a patient has no other family to help, he or she might be tempted to name someone who offers assistance to have complete power of attorney. In this scenario, all financial and legal issues are then controlled by this designee, who could steal funds and property. This level of complete access to your legal and monetary control should be reserved for the most trusted friend or relative.

Do Not Resuscitate (DNR)

A Do-Not-Resuscitate order is exactly what it says and no more. In the event that the patient suffers a cardiac arrest (outside surgery or the cardiac catheterization lab, generally), no resuscitative measures will be taken: no chest compressions, no ventilation, and no drugs. For patients with a reasonable chance of recovery, because they are young, in good general condition, or the cause of their cardiac arrest is reversible, resuscitation is a reasonable choice. Comparing two cardiac arrests, a child has a better chance of a full life after a cold-water drowning than an older adult with existing health problems who suffers multiple injuries and blood loss in a car crash.

For patients who have terminal diseases, however, making the decision about resuscitation is absolutely essential: if a patient already has a terminal disease, resuscitation will, at best, return him to his condition just prior to the arrest. More often, return of a beating heart will include worsening of existing conditions, plus other catastrophic medical issues, such as kidney failure or ventilator dependence.

When a patient has not made those decisions beforehand, loved ones will be asked to answer the question to resuscitate or not. The answer should consider the quality of life possible if resuscitation is chosen and successful.

What Happens During Cardiac Resuscitation?

For those who don't understand the processes, resuscitation of someone in a cardiac arrest is not a dignified and gentle process. Let me offer some brutal details. First, breathing is managed by a device that pushes air down the airway into the lungs, but also into the stomach. It's not uncommon that stomach contents are regurgitated then forced into the lungs during manual ventilation, setting up pneumonia if the arrest is survived. Eventually a tube is placed through the mouth or nose into the trachea to protect the airway from this regurgitation and to provide a more stable ventilation path; this tube will be connected to a ventilator machine. Chest compressions provide external force to push blood out of the heart to critical organs, but this can cause rib fractures that will be extremely painful during recovery and may add to the risk of pneumonia. Also, broken ribs may puncture the lungs or the heart. Blood flow from chest compressions is intended to save the brain, the heart, the lungs, and then the kidneys before other organ systems, such as the digestive tract, but the kidneys are the last of the critical organs to receive oxygenation with low blood pressure of compressions, so failure of blood filtration may result. Depending on the time that has elapsed before chest compressions are begun, the brain may be irreversibly damaged by lack of oxygen. Intravenous routes for drugs and fluid are accessed, sometimes through upper chest, neck, or femoral sites rather than arms. Electrical shock may be used to allow the heart to return to a pulsing rhythm.

From an outsider's viewpoint, resuscitation may appear ghastly and violent. The processes, while brutal in appearance, are a well-researched sequence of tasks shown to maximize return of spontaneous pulse and breathing. Unfortunately, it doesn't always work successfully. Loved ones who have to make decisions regarding whether this is to happen must realize the chances of survival and the risk of failure, even if a pulse returns.

No one likes to talk about dying, but decisions made by a patient beforehand can remove many doubts and regrets of family members who may have to make those decisions later.

Picking a Legal Healthcare Advocate

Several rules dictate who cannot be a legal healthcare advocate, disqualifying anyone under the age of 18; any direct healthcare provider; an employee of your healthcare provider unless this person is a spouse or close relative; and anyone who owns and/or operates a healthcare facility in which you are a patient unless this person is a spouse or close relative.

Questions you should consider when deciding on a healthcare agent include:

- Does this person know your wishes and is he willing to speak on your behalf in a medical emergency, even in the face of adversity or conflict?
- Do you trust this person with your life?
- Does this person live nearby to be able to state your wishes in person when necessary?
- Is this person someone who will be available well into the future for you?

You need to make sure this person has copies of your legal documents, and that family members know who this healthcare agent is and what decisions can be made by him or her.

Next, you should take time to consider your current state of health, and what conditions might be worse to survive than death itself. For example, if you can no longer interact with family or the world around you, such as after a severe stroke, would you want the decision to be made to provide all available care to continue your life, or would you want to avoid treatments to prolong your life? Do you want to be dependent on ventilation machines, kidney dialysis, or feeding tubes in order to live? Does it depend on whether the condition is deemed irreversible? What if you are in uncontrollable pain?

The best answers to these questions are decided ahead of any critical illnesses; if they are not made, however, they will fall upon the patient's healthcare agent—that advocate who can make choices for the patient.

CHAPTER 13

Hospice

Americans hesitate to discuss decisions about healthcare for a variety of reasons, and death is sometimes viewed as taboo. My parents used to say they didn't want to talk about those things, but I finally got them to complete their wills. Hospice care is a logical progression as patients move away from successful treatment of their conditions, but family members worry, "I don't want Dad to think we're giving up on him," or "I don't want all of Mom's care to be stopped."

Neither perception of hospice is correct. Hospice care has a variety of advantages for patients who suffer terminal diseases or conditions, and for their families.

- Hospice offers palliative care—care of symptoms and pain—not curative treatment of the terminal illness.
- The focus is quality of life rather than staying alive.
- Care offers comfort and dignity for dying patients and their loved ones.
- Medical, emotional, spiritual, and practical-care support is available to the patient and family.

- Hospice views both life and death as normal processes, but the care neither hastens nor postpones death.

A patient or family doesn't have to wait for a doctor to bring up entering a hospice program. It's available to any patient with a life-limiting illness or condition, usually with a life expectancy of less than six months. However, should a patient live longer than the six-month time, the patient is simply re-enrolled in the program. If a patient shows signs of recovery, such as cancer in remission, patients can be discharged to return to aggressive medical therapy or to return to their daily lives, and can be returned to hospice care at a later date if necessary.

Patients who have Medicare will sign a form electing Medicare Hospice benefit, which affects their Medicare coverage. Medicare Hospice Benefit covers the full scope of medical and support services for a life-limiting disease and almost all aspects of hospice care with little expense to the family.

Pain Management

Management of pain is a significant function of hospice care. Relief of physical pain is managed with medications as necessary, but emotional support and religious assistance are also available.

The goal of hospice is not to medicate a patient into oblivion so he or she cannot talk or know what is happening: it is to find balance between pain control and being alert. Some families, or even unfamiliar healthcare providers, may be alarmed at the high doses of pain medications a patient can take and still be fully functional and mentally alert. Addiction is not a concern when a patient is suffering a terminal condition; where there is real pain being treated, there is a correct chemical absorption of pain medication without risk for addiction. Tolerance and necessary dosage increases might be necessary, but this is an expected course for lengthy therapy as well.

A great resource about hospice care is:

http://www.hospicenet.org/index.html .

One misconception about hospice is that a patient will no longer receive any treatment at all. Hospice care is not "giving up" treatment for non-terminal diseases or conditions. A patient with brain cancer, for example, will still be treated for a broken arm because the expectation is that the patient will recover from the injury. A patient with lung cancer who develops pneumonia might not receive aggressive treatment if not expected to recover from the infection due to progression of the cancer. In either case, the goal is of treatment is to make the patient comfortable, and to optimize the quality of her life.

My Mother's Final Weeks

Hospice cared for my mother during her very last days, and those nurses and the other staff made her death a little bit less painful.

In 2005, my mother had been suffering with emphysema for ten years. She was slowly going downhill until she could barely care for herself and the household she'd proudly maintained for 50 years with my father. In her last hospitalization, I came to her ICU room in the middle of the night, having just flown in. Late in the night, she turned away from me and said, "Let's go." When I asked her where she wanted to go, she turned to me and shook her head adamantly, then turned back to where there was no one visible to me and repeated, "Let's go." I knew her time to leave us was near.

A few nights later, she suffered a sudden onset of pulmonary edema—

fluid on her lungs—which made it difficult for her to breathe. After much intervention, she was finally resting when I talked to my father and sister about choosing hospice for her. Dad told me he didn't want her to think we'd given up on her. Fortunately, the hospice intake coordinator who came to talk with him presented hospice care as positive, both for Mom and for us. She was transported to an inpatient facility because we doubted there was time to set up care at home before she died, and the hospice staff took such wonderful care of us all—allowing us to stay around the clock, providing a place to sleep, snacks, and a place to escape for short intervals. What I found most heartfelt was that we were allowed to be a part of directing her care, even after my mother apparently had a stroke and could no longer communicate with us.

Her death was peaceful and in the company of those of us who loved her. While we miss her, I wouldn't ask her back into the agony she'd suffered before. Hospice made letting go of her just a little easier.

CHAPTER 14

Organ Donation

During the crisis of emergency and imminent death of their loved one, families are often faced with the choice regarding organ donation. These discussions are held with compassionate healthcare providers like Mia Hunter, RN, BSN, a Donation Clinical Specialist for LifeGift, (http://www.lifegift.org). Established in 1987, LifeGift is a not-for-profit organ procurement organization that recovers organs and tissue for individuals needing transplants in 109 Texas counties in North, Southeast, and West Texas. All organ donation is regulated by UNOS, the United Network for Organ Sharing, where coordination of donors and recipients is managed.

Did You Know?

- More than 113,858 patients are on the national organ transplant waiting list. More than eight patients a day are added to that waiting list, according to Mia Hunter of LifeGift. Each day, 18 people die because the organs they need are not available.
- One healthy donor can provide critical organs to save the lives of

up to eight people; many more can be helped with non-critical organs and tissue. There were 2,263 transplants in January 2012, from 1,105 donors.

- Organs you can donate: heart, kidneys, pancreas, lungs, liver, and intestines.
- Tissue you can donate: cornea, skin, bone marrow, heart valves, and connective tissue.
- To be transplanted, organs must receive oxygenated blood until they are removed from the body of the donor. Therefore, it may be necessary for the patient to remain on a ventilator until organs are retrieved..
- If a patient is older or seriously ill, then organs or tissue may not be suitable for transplant. Donation coordinators evaluate the options at or near the time of death.
- The body of an organ donor can still be shown and buried after death.
- Most donation referrals or "clinical triggers" are based on the following: the patient has suffered a brain injury (trauma, stroke, anoxic injury such as drowning), is on a ventilator, and has a Glasgow Coma Scale of 5 or less without sedation.
- Once a patient meets these criteria, the hospital staff has one hour to call to an organ coordinator to evaluate the case and to coordinate donation.
- Organ donation is not a consideration while the medical team is trying to save the life of the patient. Donation is only considered

> Websites of interest:
>
> *http://www.lifegift.org*
> *http://www.donatelifeamerica.net*

after a patient has suffered brain death or when death is imminent.

If being an organ or tissue donor is part of your wishes, it is necessary that you register to donate, but also that your family or legal guardians know. Hospitals and organ banks will ask survivors to give their permission for donation, regardless of registration. Texas has passed a law stating that any person who has registered has given "first-person consent" to donate that cannot be revoked by family members. However, in other states, family members can still refuse to abide by the wishes of the patient to donate, just like not following a DNR request for their loved one. Knowing ahead of time that a patient wishes to donate can make this less a surprise, leaving time to learn about donation processes and helping make the decision less emotional.

A close friend of mine lost his sister to a massive stroke, but she was an organ donor. Even in his grief over her death, he found solace that her donation helped many others. Here is his story:

September 4, 2008, was a horrible day. My brother-in-law called to tell me that my sister Julie, 52, had suffered a massive stroke while vacationing in San Diego. She was brain dead but on a respirator for two reasons. First, the respirator would keep Julie's body alive so that the family could make their way to San Diego to say goodbye, and second, so that her organs could be retrieved for donation. Organ donation!? What did that mean? He explained that Julie had elected to be an organ donor. I had to contemplate that. I did not know of my sister's decision to be an organ donor. I was struggling to come to terms with her death, and now I had to absorb an organ harvest. The information was unsettling, to say the least.

At first I was so busy with the logistics of family notification, I did not have time to really consider what was about to happen. My sister had just died. I was not going to be able to go to San Diego to tell her goodbye. I was not going to be able to go to the funeral. I was grieving. But I was also remembering Julie and her life.

In life, Julie was a generous person with a kind and giving heart. In death, she would continue her legacy. Her death saved four lives and assisted over sixty others. WOW! At that moment I ceased grieving for my lost sister and began rejoicing for the sixty-plus people I was now connected to through Julie. I will never know the people Julie's death impacted, but I feel a connection with them. I take comfort in the fact I may have been in the airport and stood in line with the person who received Julie's heart, or exchanged pleasantries with the person who received a kidney, or smiled at someone who had received Julie's corneas and now their eyes light up the same way Julie's did.

Since Julie's death I have done a little research on organ donation, and I have been amazed to learn how many organs are harvested and how they are used. My entire perspective on organ donation has changed.

SECTION IV

MEDICATIONS

CHAPTER 15

Know Your Medications

One study estimates that 83% of American adults take at least one medication per day, and 29% take five or more. According to data provided by the PRIME Institute for Families USA, prescriptions for the elderly have risen from 19.6 per year in 1992 to 38.5 per year in 2010. This huge increase may be due to the development of more specific drugs to treat diseases. However, in some cases this is also part of what healthcare providers call "polypharmacy," where a patient is given a medication to treat one disease process, then another to treat the side effects of the first drug, and then another to treat side effects of the second drug, and so on.

The Food and Drug Administration must approve any medication, whether prescription or over-the-counter (OTC), but lack of approval

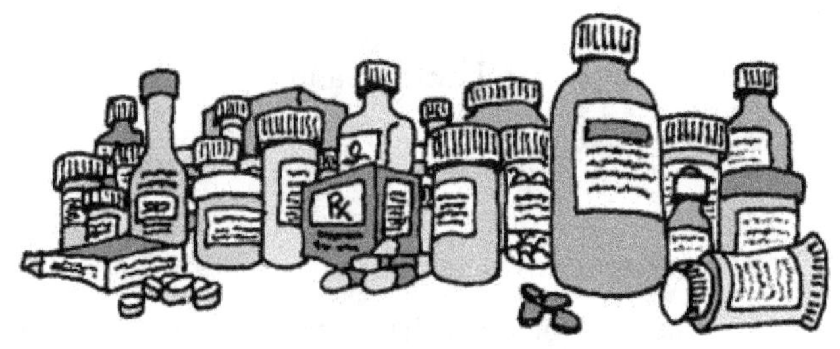

When our medicine cabinets runneth over

doesn't keep a "drug" from being sold. Many of the pills advertised on television for weight loss or other ailments clearly, but in tiny print, state that the FDA has not approved them, meaning that their actual effectiveness and/or safety may be an issue.

With medicine cabinets full of prescription and non-prescription drugs, it's more important than ever to understand what each medication is expected to do, how it may interact with other drugs being taken, and how to correctly take the proper dose.

Read the label and follow the dosing directions. Pharmacists are qualified to discuss your questions about any medication. Almost all pharmacies have a policy to ask if you need to talk with the pharmacist or if you've taken a certain medication before. Ask questions.

Listing and Understanding Medications

As a patient, you need to carry a list of all medications that you take regularly, whether prescribed or over-the-counter. More importantly, you need to understand:

- The trade and generic name for each medication,
- Why it is prescribed and the intended goal,
- How often to take it,
- When to stop taking it,
- What not to eat or drink with it, and
- When to not take it at all.

Many healthcare providers don't take the time to provide details about dietary limitations for most drugs, for example, perhaps assuming that the pharmacist will address these issues. Or they may give this information for one type of medication, but not another. A provider may tell one patient not to eat foods with Vitamin K when taking Coumadin (warfarin), but overlook telling another patient who takes Cordarone (amiodarone) not to consume grapefruit juice because it reduces the effectiveness of the medication. A physician might prescribe nitroglycerine for chest pain but neglect to tell the patient to sit down before taking it because it can decrease blood pressure enough to cause fainting.

Your list of medications should include both the trade/brand name and the generic name of each drug. The brand name is a trademarked name, such as Tylenol, Motrin, or Coumadin. The generic name is the general name for a drug that multiple manufacturers may produce. The generic name of Tylenol is acetaminophen, and it is produced by six other companies, such as Perrigo and Ranbaxy, as store or "generic" brands.

Knowing both the trade and generic name of your drugs can help prevent a duplication error when one provider prescribes Ativan and another prescribes lorazepam, which is the same drug. Also, knowing that Lortab or Norco is a combination of hydrocodone and acetaminophen can help you understand why taking Tylenol (acetaminophen) is duplicating a drug that can be toxic when taken in too high a dose.

What Does the Drug Do?

Some medications have multiple actions, such as aspirin, which may be used to treat fever or minor pain, to prevent blood clots, or to treat patients having a heart attack. Viagra (sildenafil) was originally used in hospitals to lower critically high blood pressure by dilating blood vessels. It later became a specialty drug to treat erectile dysfunction. A number of drugs are used for completely different reasons. Cymbalta, made by Eli Lilly, was approved by the FDA to treat depression (2004), diabetic nerve pain (2004), generalized anxiety disorder (2007), fibromyalgia (2008), and has been approved in Europe, but not the U.S., for urinary stress incontinence (Russell, 2008).

Other drugs are used to treat similar diseases. Enbrel, made by Amgen, is approved for rheumatoid arthritis, psoriasis, and ankylosing spondylitis (a chronic, painful condition of bone joints including the spine). Lyrica, a Pfizer pain medication for fibromyalgia, is also approved for other chronic conditions, such as nerve pain and partial seizures. Divalproex is approved for epilepsy, but is also used to treat bipolar manic episodes, and to prevent chronic migraine headaches. The drug amitriptyline is an antidepressant that is sometimes prescribed for patients with sleeping disorders and chronic pain syndromes. Benadryl (diphenhydramine) is a common antihistamine that induces drowsiness, so it is also an ingredient in over-the-counter sleep aids, such as Tylenol PM.

Dosing Instructions

It is said that the difference between a drug and a poison is just the

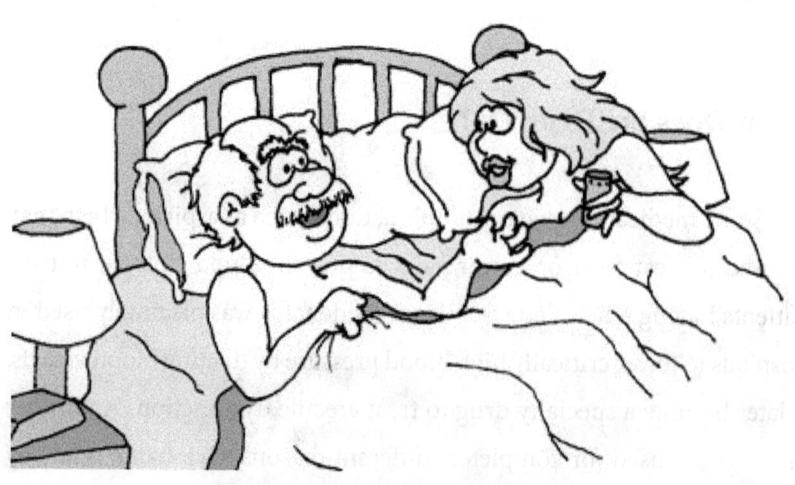

One Works good, so let's try three!

dose. Patients need to be aware of how much to take of each medication. Prescription drugs come with clear dosing directions on the label, yet some patients elect not to follow instructions. Over-the-counter drugs are incorrectly dosed just as often. For some, the rationale is, if two will help a headache, three or four will work better. Not only is this incorrect logic; it can kill you.

One of the most common drugs patients take more than recommended is acetaminophen (Tylenol). This may be intentional because two tablets don't cure the pain, so the patient takes a greater quantity, or takes the drug more often than recommended. It could be accidental because the patient does not know that a prescription drug, such as Norco or Vicodin, contains acetaminophen as well as a narcotic. However, acetaminophen, like most other drugs, does not work better at higher-than-recommended dosages. Taking more does not increase the effectiveness, and too much can be fatal.

Appropriate concentrations for infants and children are also critical. Who would think that infant Tylenol (acetaminophen) drops are far more concentrated than children's drops, and thus the amount given is very different? Infant doses contain 160 milligrams per milliliter, while children's liquid has only 100 milligrams per milliliter. The difference is the amount of liquid an infant or child can effectively swallow. However, a mother of children taking both formulas may treat the drugs as interchangeable when they are not, thus overdosing a toddler with infant drops.

Another reason patients may take a wrong dose of medication is prescription changes. When the healthcare provider increases the dose, he may agree the smaller dose can be doubled until the purchased medication is gone to prevent waste; however, when the new strength prescription is filled, the patient may forget that now only one is needed.

Understanding the purpose and function of each medication is vital.

You might take both Lasix and Accupril for high blood pressure. Each medication works differently to achieve the desired effect. Often, drugs are paired to create a certain response because one drug depletes what is replaced by another. Lasix (furosemide) is almost always paired with potassium chloride replacement because it depletes potassium when the diuretic causes the body to remove water.

Another potential problem is when doctors overlook the inactive ingredients of a drug. A woman who has had diabetes for a long time developed acid reflux. She was referred to a specialist, who gave her samples of a new drug, Dexilant. In the ten days she took this, her blood sugars were drastically high and out of control. Because she had samples and no package insert, research about the drug was necessary. Two of the first three ingredients were sugar spheres and sucrose! When she told the prescribing doctor this information, he argued that the drug couldn't possibly make her blood sugar go up. Despite data from the manufacturer's drug insert and the drug website stating this was possible, the prescribing doctor refused to acknowledge that the drug had a negative impact on her health.

How and When Do I Take It?

When a prescription states the drug should be taken three or four times a day, you should confirm with the pharmacist whether this means you might need to wake from sleep to take a night dose. Some over-the-counter drugs for cold and flu symptoms can be taken as often as every four hours, so their relief may wear off during the night. However, most prescription medications taken for more than one month are generally formulated to last eight to twelve hours, making scheduling doses simpler.

Some drugs can be taken without regard to timing of meals. Others must be taken on an empty stomach or after a meal. Some drugs cannot be taken with other drugs that alter the acidity of the stomach, or with certain types of food or juice. Coumadin, for example, is frequently prescribed for evening dosing. Thyroid medications are generally prescribed to be taken on an empty stomach in the morning. Some come as "sprinkle" capsules, which may be swallowed whole or opened and sprinkled onto a teaspoon of soft, cool food, such as applesauce or pudding. Before crushing other tablets that are very large, this should be discussed with a pharmacist. Extended-release formulas should never be crushed or opened as splitting a capsule will destroy the enteric coating designed to release the medication into your system gradually.

Did I Take It?

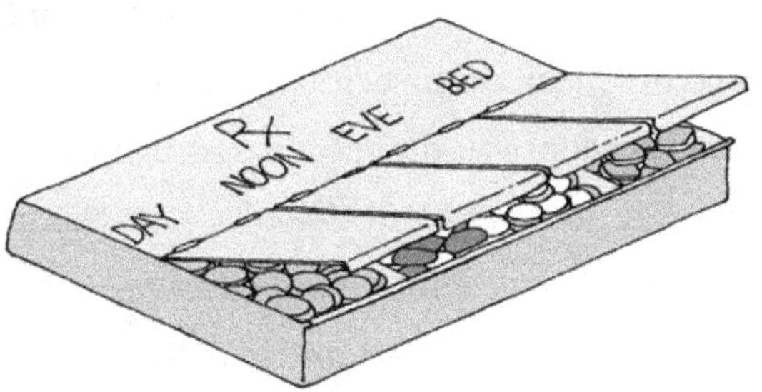

Patients who take a number of drugs at different times of the day should use a drug organizer. While it takes time to set up daily or weekly, knowing by looking that you have taken morning meds, or not yet taken lunch meds, can make scheduling and transporting them more convenient. Be sure to keep medication bottles with prescribing information. For daily, weekly, or monthly medication, a calendar chart can be useful.

Take as Directed

Prescription medications need to be taken as the healthcare provider directs. Overuse of a drug can be as detrimental as not taking it. For example, antibiotic use needs to be limited to those bacterial infections the body cannot fight on its own, such as a bacterial pneumonia or a joint bursitis. They should not be prescribed for a cold (which is often viral, not bacterial), or a simple laceration without signs of infection. If antibiotics are not indicated, do not demand them from your healthcare provider. If they are prescribed, finish them as directed.

When Not to Take a Medication as Prescribed

Knowing when not to take a medication is just as important as when and how you should. You should know the parameters for the expected effects of a medication, such as blood pressure, heart rate, or blood sugar. If your response to the medication falls outside the norm, call your healthcare provider. Many side effects, such as unintentional movement, blurred vision, and fainting are early signs of potentially life-threatening reactions and need to be reported immediately.

One other time when medications may not perform as expected is when using patch medications (dermal medication delivery, such as blood pressure regulation, smoking cessation, or pain control). Continued application during a fever can cause an overdose or alter the duration of effectiveness.

Sample Medication and History List

Medications		
Date Prescribed	**Brand/generic name/ dose/instructions**	**Reason Taken**
Aug 2010	Prinivil (lisinopril) 20 mg twice a day	High blood pressure
Allergies		
	Brand/generic name	**Reaction**
Medication	Codeine	Vomiting
Food	Peanuts	Difficulty breathing
	Seafood	Vomiting, Swelling
Environmental	Latex	Rash, hives
Medical History		
Current Illnesses/ Conditions	High blood pressure	
Previous Illnesses	Pneumonia 2003	
Surgeries	Appendectomy 1993	
Hospitalizations	Pneumonia 2003 Appendicitis 1993 Fractured leg 1974	

CHAPTER 16

Buying Medications

Trade Name Versus Generic: What's the Difference?

A trade or brand name of a drug is exclusive to a particular manufacturer, has a specific formula, and early in its licensing is ineligible for generic formulas. Tylenol is a trade name for the generic drug acetaminophen, which is also manufactured and marketed by other companies as a generic. Plavix, produced by Bristol-Myers Squibb/Sanofi Pharmaceuticals Partnership is a trade name for the generic drug clopidogrel, for which the patent has just expired, making it eligible for generic equivalent. Pradaxa (dabagatran) by Boehringer Ingelheim, is still available only as a trade-name.

In comparing brand-name drugs to generic drugs, equivalent is the key. A generic drug contains the same active ingredient(s) as the brand-name medication, but it will not necessarily be identical in the non-essential formula. Per studies related by the Food and Drug Administration, the essential content (active ingredient) may vary as much as 3.5%. That small variation may be the very amount that causes a drug to be ineffective, or too effective, in its treatment. For blood pressure control, a generic might not bring the pressure into a target range, or it could cause the blood pressure to be too low.

Any generic drug modeled after a single brand-name drug (the reference) must perform approximately the same in the body as the brand name drug. There may be a slight, but usually not medically important,

> Website for the Food and Drug Administration
>
> *http://www.fda.gov/Drugs/ResourcesForYou/Consumers/BuyingUsingMedicineSafely/UnderstandingGenericDrugs/ucm167991.htm*

level of natural variability, just as there slight variation in performance from one batch of brand-name drug to the next. The Food and Drug Administration details these variations and regulations on its website.

What this means to you is that a change to a generic drug may make no difference at all in the effectiveness of the drug you take, and may mean a significant savings. However, for a small group of individuals, generic drugs do not perform as expected. You should be aware of this potential, as changes may be made without your knowledge, such as when you are in the hospital, or if your healthcare is provided within a large system, such as the Veteran's Administration.

It is your right to have a formula that performs to expectations, though this may mean you have to continue to pay for a trade-name medication instead of the cheaper generic formula.

Formulary

A formulary is a list of approved drugs, usually issued by an insurance company, to control costs of prescriptions for which it has a price agreement or preferred generic-formula choice. Although this is not always an issue, formulary limitation can impact the medications prescribed to a patient, forcing a change. For example, a formulary might cover warfarin in a generic formula with a patient copay of $10, but the copay for the brand name Coumadin is $20. For Ranexa (which has no generic equivalent), the copay might be $40 or more. One of the newest drug anticoagulant drugs, Pradaxa, is not offered at all by many insurance formularies. You may choose to pay more for uncovered medications for a variety of reasons, but may not be able to afford to do so. In another case, one blood-pressure medication may be substituted with a preferred drug. For example, metoprolol (Lopressor or Toprol-XL) might be mandated instead of atenolol (Tenormin). However, a patient may find that the substituted drug is not effective in lowering blood pressure to acceptable levels.

Formulary changes are supposed to be in the patient's favor financially, but the change in drug may fail to treat a condition. You need to know what the goal of a medicine is in order to decide whether it is doing its job.

When a particular medication is substituted by a formulary, it is important to remember that the drug must be effective for the patient. If a medication does not perform as expected, your physician may request an exclusion to allow you to receive a non-formulary medicine, often at the reduced cost.

Choosing a Pharmacy

Today, you have a wide variety of choices in pharmaceutical services, but it pays to choose wisely. First, of course, a pharmacy must participate in your prescription coverage program. There are also pharmacies that offer a basic list of drugs at deeply discounted prices for those without insurance who may need medications.

Second, although a hometown pharmacy may have staff that knows its customers individually, it's more important that the pharmacist has access to more than your name to fill a prescription. With electronic health records becoming more readily available, a pharmacist should be able to compare drugs prescribed to those already being taken being taken and to those a patient should not take. As mentioned before, physicians may not take the time to look up past medications and allergies, so a competent pharmacist should—and so should you.

Third, larger-chain pharmacies are beginning to compete for business in non-drug sales as well, offering exclusive sales to member cardholders or discounts for the rest of the year after spending a certain amount. In some cases, these discounts can make shopping for those items at the pharmacy more convenient than at a grocery store. Chain stores may offer a huge variety of items from photographic services to food.

No matter where you have your prescription filled, it is your responsibility to check the drug to make sure it was the correct medication and the correct dosage. As a paramedic, I used to transport a young man for dialysis three times a week. He had been rendered comatose by the wrong medication. He was supposed to receive a drug for a stomach ailment; instead, his pharmacy gave him a sound-alike drug for high blood sugar in non-insulin-dependent diabetics. The end result was a 23-year-old man who had no cognitive brain function because his blood sugar had been driven down after three days of taking the wrong drug. Perhaps this tragedy could have been avoided if the patient had asked the pharmacist for information about the intended effects of the prescription, or had known what drug he was expecting.

Another way you can safeguard your health is to use a single pharmacy to fill prescribed medications. In my experience, a doctor will write a prescription for a new drug without being fully aware of previously prescribed medicines or allergies, and without regard to prescribed medications from other providers. Most chain stores now have computerized records allowing the pharmacist to cross-reference to all other prescribed medications and allergies, and to assess the incompatibility of a new medication to others, though this is part of the health information technology programs that are part of the healthcare bill. Another advantage to using a national chain is being able to refill medications from any other location if needed, making obtaining medications while traveling easier.

International and Internet Pharmaceutical Purchases

Occasionally a physician will follow research on new drugs from other countries and find that a particular patient may benefit from one, but the FDA has not yet approved its use. If the medication is available from legitimate sources in Canada or a European country, a physician may convince the patient to procure it through online sources, or where it is feasible to travel outside the United States to obtain it. However, if you attempt to do this on your own, you must be very careful because some companies are only interested in making a profit with no concern about what is being sold. The counterfeit pharmaceutical business is worth millions.

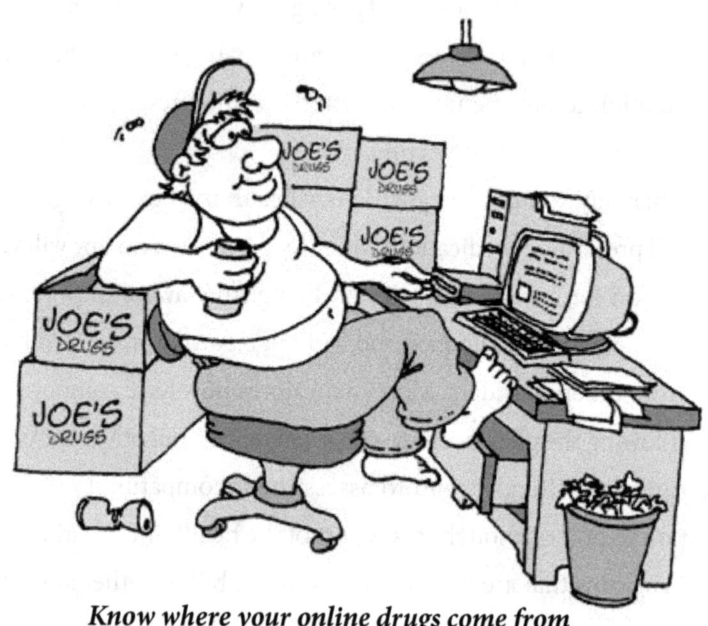

Know where your online drugs come from

Some years ago, as recommended by her lung specialist, I investigated and purchased for my mother an inhaled respiratory medication that was expected to receive FDA approval (as Spiriva) within the next six months. The purchase was made from a Canadian company the doctor had done business with previously, so he felt it was reliable. However, the drug was also available from many sources I would not have considered to be trustworthy.

There is a huge online market for narcotics, antibiotics, and even medications for erectile dysfunction. You may be tempted to buy these drugs online instead of getting them legitimately in the United States because of cost, embarrassment of going to the doctor, or unprescribed use, but this practice can be dangerous. According to the World Health Organization, in over 50% of cases, medicines purchased over the Internet from sites that conceal their physical addresses are counterfeit (WHO, 2010b). This is a risk you should not take, even if it seems like it will save you a lot of money.

When a drug is counterfeit, it may contain more, less, or completely different substances that don't correctly treat a condition. These medications may have ingredients that cause serious or fatal side effects when used with legitimate medications. Some contain poisonous substances, such as lead or arsenic. Worse still, you may have purchased a medication without consulting a healthcare provider to see if it is even necessary. Incorrect treatment can lead to dangerous complications.

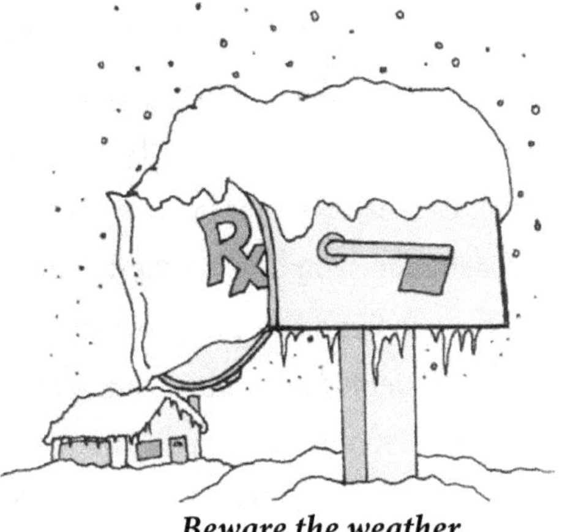

Beware the weather, if you receive drugs by mail

Medication Shipping

A number of pharmaceutical insurance companies use a discounted direct mail service for cost-savings and convenience of their patients. However, as a patient, you should consider more than convenience. Both heat and cold can affect potency of medications, making them more or less potent than expected. An envelope sitting in an outdoor mailbox all day in the heat of summer, or in a winter snowstorm, could put you at risk.

If you use a mail-order prescription service, you might consider getting a post office box that can be the designated receiving point for your medications. However, even that step cannot prevent your packages being in uncontrolled temperatures during transit.

Over-the-Counter (OTC) Drugs

Many people consider all medicines purchased over the counter to be safe, but drugs like aspirin, acetaminophen, ibuprofen, and naproxen, to name a few, can interact with any prescription medications you may take. For example, aspirin can be taken occasionally for mild pain or fever, daily in a small dose for prevention of cardiovascular disease, as needed or for sudden symptoms of chest pain. However, taking aspirin regularly without telling a healthcare provider could result in uncontrolled bleeding when a patient is prescribed Coumadin or Plavix.

Another consideration is that not all pills or liquids in a pharmacy are approved by the FDA. Several weight-loss aids have been recalled for contamination or for failure to list all ingredients. Talk to your pharmacist before buying.

Herbs or supplements used in complementary or alternative medicine (CAM) are often not mentioned to healthcare providers. Supplements and herbs can have a real effect on the body but can also result in dangerous interactions with other medications. Use of complimentary therapies should be carefully coordinated with a healthcare provider who knows what they are, and supplements should be purchased through reliable dealers and reputable manufacturers.

The National Center for Complementary and Alternative Medicine (which is part of the National Institutes of Health) has a website with news about research, clinical trials, health information, and a detailed explanation of the herbs and other supplements commonly used in alternative medicine. *http://nccam.nih.gov*

A list published in September 2010 of *Consumer Reports* magazine lists the following supplements as safe for use: calcium, fish oil, cranberry, glucosamine sulfate, lactase, lactobacillus, psyllium, pygeum, SAMe, St. John's wort, and vitamin D. The same article suggests that one should never use the following without the specific expertise of a caregiver familiar with complimentary or alternative medicine (CAM): aconite, bitter orange, chaparral, colloidal silver, coltsfoot, comfrey, country mallow, germanium, greater celandine, kava, lobelia, and yohimbe (*Consumer Reports*, 2010).

Other substances you should discuss with your healthcare provider before using include aloe vera juice, ephedra, ginger, ginkgo biloba, saw palmetto, and valerian.

The U.S. Pharmacopeia also provides information about supplements and nutraceuticals, and verifies specific brand names of products, such as fish oil. This means that the products are regularly tested for quality, and for contaminants, such as mercury. Their website is *http://www.USP.org*

It's not the intention of this book to advise for or against the use of alternative medicines; rather, I'd like to stress their safe use. Be sure to list them as medications when making a list for your healthcare provider. Providers who are familiar with them can provide safe directions for the purchase and use of complementary and alternative supplements.

CHAPTER 17

Medication Challenges

Medication Allergies

Many people think that a medication is causing an allergic reaction when it causes an undesired effect, such as nausea and vomiting. However, when a healthcare provider asks you about drug allergies, you need to name true allergy symptoms, such as difficulty breathing; swelling of the lips, mouth, and throat; or a severe rash; list medications you don't tolerate well (but are not allergic to) and their reactions, too.

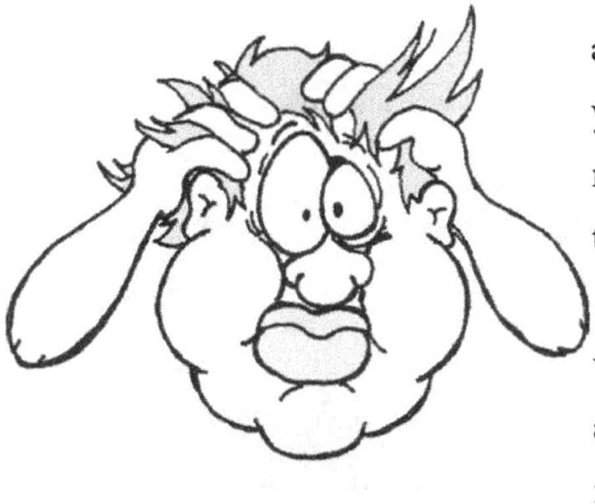

Allergies might include Facial Swelling, Itching or Difficulty Breathing

While you need to discuss with your healthcare provider any medication that causes itching or vomiting, there is a clear difference between an allergic reaction and a potentially life-threatening anaphylactic reaction. Any life-threatening reaction, such as swelling of the face, tongue and throat, or drop in blood pressure must be communicated to your healthcare provider. Peanuts, penicillin, or latex in gloves and other medical devices can cause critical or fatal allergic reactions. Avoidance is not a matter of being polite. It is essential to your health and needs to be expressed without hesitation.

Drug Errors

Patients who are well versed in their medication needs are less likely to be victims of drug errors. When admitted to a hospital, you should know whether your admission is "for observation" or a full admit. Insurance representatives may advise you to bring your own drugs to the hospital when you are admitted for a 23-hour observation. Taking your own medications can lead to confusion as to which drugs have been taken, and may also lead to your receiving duplicate medications. If so directed, take your medications in their prescription bottles to the hospital, and discuss them with the nursing staff to help alleviate any discrepancy.

Another fact to remember is that drugs given to a patient in the hospital often differ in appearance due a difference in manufacturer or dose. For cost control, combination drugs may not be available, so each of the component drugs is given instead. Exforge for blood pressure might not be available, so separate amlodipine and valsartan would be given instead.

You have the right to question all medications, and you also have the right to refuse to take any if the answers are unsatisfactory with regard to type, dose, or duplication. Your nursing provider wants to make sure you are getting correct medications, so the more you know about what you take, the better prepared you will be to discuss the matter.

Drug Recalls

Anyone who buys medications should also pay attention to announcements of recalls, which are covered by the news media. Last year, a recall of Tylenol Extra Strength was made due to identification of an "odd odor." The odor reportedly did not affect the drug's performance, but the manufacturers erred on the side of caution. Another recall for Endocet (Endo Pharmaceuticals brand of oxycodone and acetaminophen) was issued because of potential incorrect dosing strength in a bottle. Previous recalls by the makers of Tylenol (McNeil, which is a Johnson & Johnson company) have involved wrong dosing concentrations and contaminants in the medication.

More recently, Novartis voluntarily recalled a number of its over-the-counter drugs because of complaints about mislabeling and broken or chipped tablets or capsules, and potential inconsistent bottle-line packaging. Novartis urged consumers to return or destroy unused products listed in its recall, including such brands as Excedrin, Bufferin, No-Doz, and Gas-X Prevention (CNN, 8 January 2012) as there was the possibility of "stray tablets, caplets, or capsules," or prescription medication being mixed with the expected packaged product. Novartis maintains that no adverse effects had been reported at the time of the recall (Novartis Consumer Health, 2012).

Awareness of recalls is necessary. Recalls are often grouped by lot number or expiration dates, both of which are on the bottles.

> Consumers can research recalls and other safety announcements on the FDA website:
>
> *http://www.fda.gov/Safety/MedWatch/SafetyInformation/default.htm*

Expiration Dates

You may be tempted to hang on to medications for a lot of reasons, such as high cost or "for next time." Drugs have an expiration date on them for a reason, and it should be heeded. Keeping a bottle of aspirin beyond expiration may result in a strong smell of vinegar, which is a sign the acetylsalicylic acid has begun breaking down into acetyl acid (vinegar).

Other medications don't offer such a clear indication of age. Don't buy 500 tablets of aspirin just because it's a "good deal" if you do not take it regularly, as it will expire before you can use it all, tempting you to take it after it's expired.

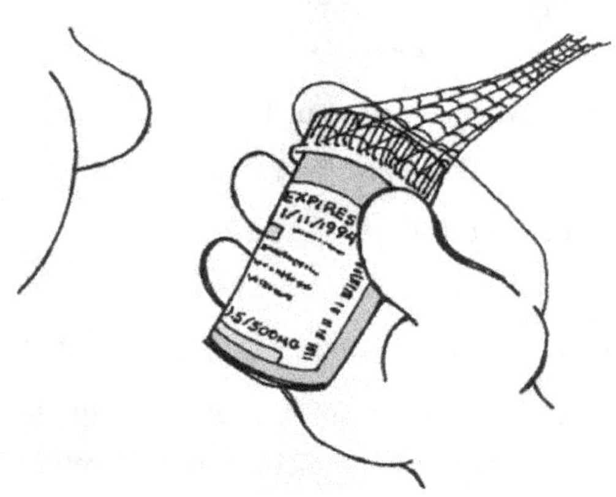

Do not take expired drugs

Medication Storage

Medications should not be stored in the bathroom where the humidity levels fluctuate, nor should they be left where temperature is uncontrolled, such as in a car. Drugs exposed to extreme environments are likely to be less effective, or even a health risk. A better choice is a hall closet, a well-ventilated cupboard in the kitchen, or a locked drawer to keep medications out of the hands and mouths of children.

Many accidental poisonings occur when a child takes medications from a purse or an unsecured area of a home where they are visiting. Medications may look like candy, making them appealing to children. Keeping medications out of the reach of children and those with cognitive difficulties can be challenging, but leaving medicines unsecured can have disastrous results. A regular adult dose can be fatal to a toddler. An adult with dementia may not understand that all medications are not theirs, or know how many they are supposed to take.

Medication Disposal

Expired or leftover drugs, such as out-of-date cold remedies or unused pain medicine may require disposal if it is leftover pain medication an expired cold remedy. Several options exist for discarding medication. The Food and Drug Administration has a list of drugs for which it recommends disposal by flushing down the toilet. The list is quite lengthy, but includes all narcotics and benzodiazepines, to keep these from being taken by someone accidentally or from being abused (FDA, 2012).

Medications that are not on this list can be disposed of in household trash after being mixed with some unpalatable substance, such as coffee grounds or used cat litter. This includes non-prescription drugs too. Another option is to return drugs to a medication-take-back program, often sponsored by pharmacies, hospitals, or other facilities. These programs are becoming increasingly popular as the number of medications increases (Office of National Drug Control Policy, 2011). Although some environmental experts are concerned that drugs are leaching into ground water sources and cause contamination, the FDA notes only trace amounts of medications in the water system, attributing the majority of this to natural body elimination and not disposal.

In all cases, before disposal, drugs should be removed from prescription containers. All labels with patient information should be destroyed or completely obliterated with permanent black marker or removed completely for privacy. Any documentation should be discarded in separate bags from the drugs, making location of them together less likely.

> If you have additional questions about disposing of your medicine, please contact the FDA at 1-888-INFO-FDA (1-888-463-6332).

Plan for Emergencies When Traveling

Especially in areas with severe winter weather, make sure you have extra medications to get through a period of isolation until the weather clears, keeping in mind that travel to a pharmacy may be limited for days after a winter storm event. Weather emergencies can isolate you at an airport for several days without any way to get refills, so make sure you have at least a week's worth of medication with you when you travel.

Travelers may call Transportation and Safety Administration (TSA) Cares toll free at 1-855-787-2227 prior to traveling with questions about screening policies, procedures and what to expect at the security checkpoint. TSA Cares will serve as an additional, dedicated resource specifically for passengers with disabilities, medical conditions or other circumstances or their loved ones who want to prepare for the screening process prior to flying. The hours of operation for the TSA Cares helpline are Monday through Friday 9 a.m.– 9 p.m. EST, excluding federal holidays. Travelers who are deaf or hard of hearing can use a relay service to contact TSA Cares or can email TSA-ContactCenter@dhs.gov.

Non-liquid or gel medications of all kinds such as solid pills, or inhalers are allowed through the security checkpoint once they have been screened. It is recommended, but not required, that your medications be labeled to assist with the screening process. For more details, see the TSA website at http://www.tsa.gov/travelers/index.shtm

More Information about Medications

There are a number of websites that you can access to read more about medications, including the U.S. Food and Drug Administration site, which features information about drugs, recalls, shortages, medical devices, vaccines, cosmetics, and even tobacco products. The site is quite comprehensive and may require several visits to view all the data you are interested in: *http://www.fda.gov/*

Another website you might investigate regarding medications is the U.S. Pharmacopeia Consumer and Patient pages at *http://www.usp.org/usp-consumers*. While the information on this site is more technical, it features information about dietary supplements and food ingredients that may be of interest.

CONCLUSION

I hope you have learned more about how to receive the best healthcare possible by being prepared and advocating for yourself or someone you care about. Some of the best healthcare treatments and facilities in the world are in the United States, but our fragmented healthcare system produces a lower life expectancy, higher rates of heart disease and cancer, and a higher rate infant mortality than other industrialized countries. Over 47 million people in the U.S. are uninsured, and millions more are under-insured.

Here are a few other staggering facts about our medical economy:

- The cost of healthcare is rising at least twice as fast as the rate of economic growth.
- Major companies and municipal governments are passing more of the cost of healthcare on to their employees.
- Many small businesses, especially in the service sector, do not provide health insurance to their employees.
- Many companies and city governments have not set aside enough money to meet healthcare obligations to retired employees.
- There is a steady rise in bankruptcies amongst individuals as well as companies due to the cost of healthcare. More than a million bankruptcies were filed in 2005 by individuals who could not afford to pay their healthcare costs.
- The cost of prescription drugs is rising even faster than the general rise in healthcare costs.

What this grim news means to you, the patient or the advocate, is that you must be in better control of your health. Start by staying healthy or becoming healthier, then ensure the healthcare you receive is effective. Follow through with the medical care regimens prescribed by your healthcare provider, speak up if you don't understand something, and remember your right to say "no" to testing and treatment that you do not want. More than ever before, it's important that you learn about your medical conditions and history, and understand your options for maintaining or improving your health.

REFERENCES

Consumer Reports. (2010). *Twelve supplements you should avoid.* Retrieved from http://www.consumerreports.org/cro/magazine-archive/2010/september/health/dangerous-supplements/supplements-to-avoid/index.htm

Food and Drug Administration. (2012). *Disposal of unused medicines: What you should know.* Retrieved from http://www.fda.gov/drugs/resourcesforyou/consumers/buyingusingmedicinesafely/ensuringsafeuseofmedicine/safedisposalofmedicines/ucm186187.htm

Novartis Consumer Health. (2012). N*ovartis Consumer Health, Inc. voluntarily recalls certain over-the-counter products in the U.S. while Novartis Group strengthens quality standards across all manufacturing sites.* Retrieved from http://www.novartis.com/newsroom/media-releases/en/2012/1575836.shtml

Online Nurse Practitioner Programs. (2012). *Physician's assistant vs. nurse practitioner: What's the difference?* Retrieved from http://onlinenursepractitionerprograms.com/nurse-practitioner-vs-physician-assistant-whats-the-difference

Perry, K. (2011). *Highlighting National Prescription Drug Take-Back Day.* Retrieved from Office of National Drug Control Policy website: http://www.whitehouse.gov/blog/2011/10/28/highlighting-national-prescription-drug-take-back-day

Russell, J. (2008). *One drug, many uses.* Good idea? Retrieved from http://www.indystar.com/article/20080629/LOCAL/806290378/One-drug-many-uses-Good-idea-

U.S. Department of Health & Human Services, Office for Civil Rights. (2012). *Health information privacy.* Retrieved from http://www.hhs.gov/ocr/privacy/

World Health Organization. (2010). *Antimicrobial resistance.* Retrieved from http://www.who.int/drugresistance/en/

World Health Organization. (2010b). *Medicines: Spurious/falsely labeled/falsified/counterfeit (SFFC) medicines.* Retrieved from http://www.who.int/mediacentre/factsheets/fs275/en

SECTION V

APPENDICES

APPENDIX A

Medication Worksheet

WHAT DO I TAKE?
WHY DO I TAKE IT?
WHEN DO I TAKE IT? ANY SPECIAL INSTRUCTIONS?
WHAT IS THE INTENDED RESULT?
WHEN SHOULD I NOT TAKE IT?
WHAT MEDICATIONS CAN I NOT TAKE AND WHY?

APPENDIX B
Medical History Form

Medications		
Date Prescribed	**Brand/generic name/ dose/instructions**	**Reason Taken**

Allergies		
	Brand/generic name	**Reaction**
Medication		
Food		
Environmental		

Medical History	
Current Illnesses/ Conditions	
Previous Illnesses	
Surgeries	
Hospitalizations	

APPENDIX C

The Healthcare Bill

The Patient Protection and Affordable Care Act was signed into law in 2010, amid much controversy. At the end of June 2012, the Supreme Court of the United States released its decision regarding the constitutionality of a portion known as the individual mandate, further dividing the gap between supporters and opponents alike. Regardless of decision, the debate continues over the mandate that will require an applicable individual and dependents to obtain and maintain minimum insurance coverage for each month starting in 2013, or else be subjected to a penalty.

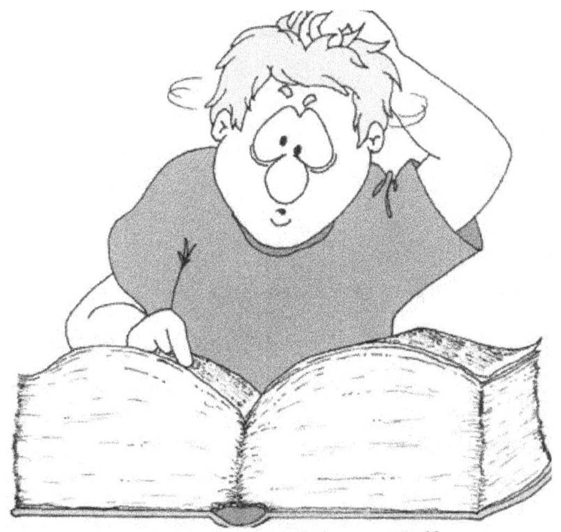

OH, the Healthcare Bill...

This bill encompasses a great deal of verbiage for hospitals, healthcare providers, and insurance companies, as well as individuals. The Act also sets into effect labeling requirements for food through restaurants and vending machines, patient-centered outcomes research, and much more. Most Americans either have been or will be affected in some way by this law. Due to its length, complexity, and inclusion of amendments to dozens of other government rulings, many people do not understand it.

A few sections of the law have been enacted, such as the requirement that insurance providers cover dependent children in a household until age 26, and that an individual cannot be excluded from coverage due to pre-existing disease or condition. For many, these two provisions offer insurance benefits that were previously too expensive or unavailable.

Another aspect under debate mandates that insurance companies will be required to use no less than 80% of the premiums paid for actual patient healthcare. Insurance companies argue that they have to use more than 20% of the premiums they collect to pay for the administrative costs of their businesses. While the premise seems valid, I suspect that the result will be an overall increase in healthcare premiums to cover that change in percentage.

As I read through this, I see multiple government agencies attempting to coordinate proof and oversight and penalties, including the Internal Revenue Service and the Secretary of Health and Human Services. Sharing information may become far more cumbersome than expected, causing delays affecting the already clogged bureaucracy.

The Act also elaborates on how "health insurance and healthcare services are a significant part of the national economy. National health spending is projected to increase from $2.5 trillion in 2009 to $4.7 trillion in 2019." Furthermore, the authors acknowledge that the Act, along with other provisions, will "add millions of new consumers to the health insurance market, increasing the supply of, and the demand for, health care services." The consequence to this, it is concluded, is that by requiring insurance coverage, the Act will "broaden the health insurance risk pool to include healthy individuals, which will lower health insurance premiums." As a nurse, I fear that this will overload the existing healthcare services before personnel and facilities can be expanded to include these added millions of people.

However, to this requirement of insurance is an exemption for "religious conscience," which states that the Act will not include "any individual for any month if such an individual has in effect an exemption ... which certifies that such an individual is a member of a recognized religious sect or division..." This section concerns me, not because of the exemption itself and how it will be put into effect, but because of the verbiage regarding "a recognized religious sect or division." Who will decide what religion is or is not "recognized" to qualify as exempt? Who gets "certified" as a member of a religion?

There are hundreds of other topics that can be debated, and I ask that you learn how these changes will affect you–both financially and medically–then get involved in the politics of supporting it or repealing it. Either way, each citizen needs to offer a voice to how healthcare changes. Contact your legislators and be active. It is time to hold responsible those few who are making healthcare reform decisions for everyone but themselves. I believe one of most important rights you have as a patient is the right to vote, so please exercise it.

APPENDIX D

Health Information Technology

Diana Cassar-Uhl, IBCLC
Reprinted with Permission

Healthcare in the United States has come a long way since the days of the hometown family doctor, one general practitioner who might address the various medical needs of an entire family throughout the life cycle, from birth to death. Today, that primary care physician/GP may be viewed as the conductor of an orchestra, coordinating a patient's care among various specialists (Gutierriez & Scheid, 2002). Healthcare Information Technology serves as the medium over which those disperse specialists can readily communicate and truly collaborate in patient care.

Healthcare Information Technology (HIT), which involves determining data needs, gathering, analyzing, and storing appropriate data, and generating reports of this data in a user-friendly format (Shi & Singh, 2012), has the potential to improve the delivery and safety of healthcare while saving costs. In 2009, the Health Information Technology for Economic and Clinical Health Act (HITECH) was incorporated as part of the American Recovery and Reinvestment Act ("stimulus"), budgeting $34 billion in incentives for healthcare professionals and hospitals that receive Medicare and Medicaid funds to incorporate meaningful use of these technologies. If these providers fail to become meaningful users of Healthcare IT by 2015, they stand to face financial penalties in the form of reduced payments for services (Consumer-Purchaser Disclosure Project, 2010).

The term meaningful use applies to specific criteria for implementation and use of Healthcare IT within the context of what Healthcare IT is designed to accomplish. These goals, or intended consequences of using Healthcare IT, have been proposed by the Centers for Medicare and Medicaid Services (CMS). They include:

- Increasing care coordination and fostering better doctor-patient communication,
- Reducing medical errors and improving patient safety,
- Supporting delivery of evidence-based care,
- Reducing disparities by recording demographic information,
- Improving quality of care, while fostering more cost-effective delivery,
- Advancing payment reform (by supplying needed data on provider performance), and
- Providing patients with their own, portable health information (Consumer-Purchaser Disclosure Project, 2010).

The criteria for defining meaningful use, set forth by Congress in the HITECH Act, are:

1. Use Electronic Health Records (EHR) certified technology in a

meaningful manner, including ePrescribing,

2. Demonstrate capability of exchanging electronic health information to improve quality, and
3. Submit information on clinical quality measures

(*Consumer-Purchaser Disclosure Project*, 2010).

Various physician organizations, such as the American Academy of Pediatrics and the American College of Cardiologists, have instituted strong encouragement to their members to meaningfully implement information technology in their practices (Center for Medicaid & Medicare Services, 2012). Meaningful use has been defined in stages, with specific goals for percentages of providers that meet the above-stated criteria by a certain time. Significant financial incentives ranging from $2000 to $18,000 are offered to Medicare and Medicaid providers that meet the standards for each stage within the proposed time frame.

Stage 1 expects that providers will collect relevant data and use it to facilitate communication between providers and to patients about conditions and care needs, and to report critical quality and public health information. Stage 2 focuses on the exchange and use of the information that was collected in Stage 1, and Stage 3 seeks to promote improvements to the entire healthcare system through patient self-management tools, a focus on decision support for high-priority conditions, and improving access to data for epidemiological purposes. Stages 1 and 2 were implemented in 2011, and Stage 3 is expected to take shape by the end of 2013 (Consumer-Purchaser Disclosure Project, 2010).

The information technology systems that are being implemented are expected to, by as early as the end of 2012, help providers communicate better with each other about patient care, reduce medical errors, cut down on paperwork, and eliminate needless duplicate screenings and tests resulting in better coordinated patient care and lower healthcare costs (Center for Medicaid & Medicare Services, 2012). The systems and their intended functions are as follows:

- The Regional Health Interchange Organization, or RHIO, is a group of organizations within a specific geographical area that share healthcare-related information electronically according to accepted healthcare information technology (HIT) standards. A RHIO typically oversees the means of information exchange among various provider settings, payers and government agencies (TechTarget, 2010). The main function of a RHIO is to provide the legal and technical capability for a healthcare provider to obtain the clinical history of a patient (Sutherland, 2005).
- Electronic Health Records (EHR) are intended to replace paper medical records, which record demographic information; health issues, diagnoses, and care plans; medical history; immunizations; and reports from labs, radiology, and other tests. The benefit of using electronic records rather than paper ones is that the information can be used in the coordination of care, quality measurement, or to reduce medical errors (Hillestad et al., 2005). The four components of a fully developed EHR system are:

    1. Collection and storage of health information on individual patients over time, where health information is defined as information pertaining to the health of an individual or healthcare provided to an individual,
    2. Immediate electronic access to person and population level information by authorized users,
    3. Provision of knowledge and decision support that enhances the quality, safety, and efficiency of patient

care, and

4. Support of efficient processes for healthcare delivery.

- ePrescribing (eRx) is the means by which a physician can electronically generate a prescription straight to a pharmacy. The various systems available for eRx also offer access to patient medical history, possible drug interactions, and contraindications to specific drugs for a patient (American Medical Association, 2012)
- Computerized Provider Order Entry (CPOE) is a system that allows healthcare providers to enter orders for prescriptions, laboratory tests, hospital admission, radiology, or other procedure orders within a hospital or ambulatory facility. Such a system replaces traditional methods of transmitting orders, such as paper, verbal, telephone, or fax. The primary purpose of CPOE is to increase safety and efficiency of medical orders that will be carried out from within a facility (Dixon & Zafar, 2009).
- Clinical Decision Support (CDS) is technology that provides guidance and feedback about a wide range of diagnostic and treatment-related information while at the same time a healthcare provider is composing the electronic orders for prescriptions, laboratory tests, or other procedures (Dixon & Zafar, 2009). The CDS systems are intended to enhance patient safety by cross-referencing such information as past diagnostic procedures and treatments, patient's weight, and other factors.

These Healthcare IT systems all stand to significantly improve the safety and efficiency of healthcare, while ultimately reducing costs. The RHIO, which will be the regional level of a National Health Information Network, serves to interconnect all of the healthcare providers across a geographical region. This interconnection will provide both a legal and a technical way to access patient information so that physicians will immediately know the diagnostic and treatment history of each patient (Sutherland, 2005). Because medical errors are often the result of an inadequate history being provided to the physician, the access to this information through the RHIO will have a positive impact on patient safety, especially in an emergency-department setting (van der Grinten, 2006). Costs will be reduced on two levels: first, because tests and procedures are less likely to be duplicated if the results of previously performed ones are readily available at the time of healthcare delivery; second, because patient outcomes will be improved overall, less money will need to be spent addressing issues that were missed (van der Grinten, 2006).

The widespread adoption of EHR systems is expected to lead to increased patient safety due to their inter-operability with other components of Healthcare IT. The intent is to make individual health records shareable between separate but interoperable systems, enabling multiple providers, such as pharmacists, physicians, and allied health workers to access patients' medical information conveniently and readily. Another initiative of EHRs is for the systems to offer evidence-based clinical decision support (CDS) that can provide reminders and best-practice guidelines for treatment (Hillestad, 2005). The success of Healthcare IT rests on the implementation of EHR systems, because all of the other components of HIT require the comprehensive data of a patient's medical records in order to be fully utilized. While the initial financial and training-time costs of setting up an EHR system can be significant, the resulting improvements in billing and the decreased need for personnel can add up to the system paying for itself within three years (Miller, et al., 2005). Additionally, as with the RHIOs, the improved outcomes that are anticipated with the widespread adoption of EHR systems will result in fewer dollars spent per patient over time.

The safety and cost implications of using the technology available for ePrescribing (eRx) are immediate and obvious. In a 2006 report entitled Preventing Medication Errors, the Institute of Medicine conservatively estimates that preventable adverse drug events (ADEs) in hospitals alone cost $3.5 billion. These ADEs are largely attributed to what are called "hand-off errors," mistakes that occur when a paper prescription is either erroneously written by the physician or misread by the pharmacist, or when a nurse or other allied healthcare provider misunderstands a verbal or written physician's order for a medication or dosage. Improved legibility and the precision of the physician's request will go a long way toward reducing the number of these preventable ADEs. In addition, eRx systems are equipped with Clinical Decision Support (CDS) elements that will alert a physician if the drug he is attempting to prescribe might interact negatively with another drug the patient is taking (perhaps prescribed by a different provider) or if the dose being prescribed is inappropriate for the patient's weight, gender, or condition. It is clear that a reduced need to correct preventable medication errors will result in reduced costs, as well as save lives and protect the health of patients.

The Computerized Provider Order Entry (CPOE) systems will have a similar, direct impact on patient safety simply because the orders themselves will be much more legible than those that are handwritten on paper. In addition, the requirement that the order be placed directly by the physician has the same effect on patient safety as the eRx system, which is that "hand-off errors" are eliminated. The Clinical Decision Support (CDS) elements of the CPOE systems are crucial to their impact in the same way these CDS real-time provisions of evidence-based protocols and clinical guidance enhance the safety of the eRx and EHR systems. Physician error is reduced, continuity of patient care is augmented, even between providers, and communication between providers is greatly improved. Better patient outcomes mean fewer dollars spent per patient. Additionally, CPOE systems allow for a facility's efficiency to be tightened up, requiring fewer staff and resulting in lower costs (Dixon & Zafar, 2009).

While the benefits to efficiency, patient safety, and costs of healthcare delivery are many with the implementation of Healthcare IT systems, there are also unintended consequences that will need to be addressed. Healthcare IT, like all information technology, will be fraught with its share of bugs due to systems being released to the market before they've been fully tested; viruses and other breaches of technical functionality, requiring immediate attention from either the vendor or the facility's IT helpdesk; potential threats to the security of personally identifiable health information and other HIPAA-protected data through the unscrupulous actions of hackers and other criminals; and the temptation for healthcare providers to use unlicensed or stolen software in an effort to save money. This is especially dangerous because it would blunt the effect of one of the most beneficial elements of Healthcare IT, the Clinical Decision Support. If software isn't appropriately purchased and registered with the vendor that created it, critical updates to protocols and alerts will not become available to those unlicensed users (Groen, Mahootian, & Goldstein, 2008). All of these technological challenges are possible, therefore, highly skilled IT staff are required, around the clock, in increasing numbers. Where some medical office staff might no longer be needed due to the increased efficiency gained by using Healthcare IT, some of those savings may need to be spent on IT staff, especially in a smaller or rural facility that isn't already equipped with such employees.

There are potential ethical challenges associated with the implementation of Health IT systems. Questions about the ownership of the data that is collected for healthcare purposes are arising: Does that data belong to the patient? To the healthcare providers who use it? To the healthcare delivery system? Who should have access to the data, and what parts of it? Related to this issue, what are the risks and benefits of the secondary use of health data? Arguably, a pronounced benefit of readily accessible health-related data is the easy ability to use it for epidemiological study, with the intended result of improving overall population health. However, could there be unintended consequences of blindly obtaining "sterilized" information from databases when compared to the current methods of subject recruitment in research? A third ethical consideration is the likelihood of exploitation or discrimination of individuals based on their health status or conditions (Groen et al., 2008). With access to a total health record, a provider would gain awareness of a patient's entire health history, regardless of whether every aspect of that history was pertinent to the concern being addressed at that visit. What measures, legal or otherwise, could be taken to protect a patient who was discriminated against based on his health history, a history that wouldn't have been available before the advent of EHRs? Will additional legislation need to be passed to account for this possibility?

In personal conversation with a member of the IT staff at Community Health Systems in Tennessee, the logistical challenges that healthcare providers may experience upon implementation of Healthcare IT systems were emphasized (B. Marinaro, personal conversation on March 24, 2012). Of particular concern to hospital staff employed by Community Health Systems is the change in workflow that accompanies the adoption of CPOEs. Because physicians are the only personnel permitted to order a procedure, more of their time is spent on such tasks, which requires other staff to assume different duties, or a change in the efficiency systems of the office/facility. The initial investments of capital and time that accompany the adoption of a Healthcare IT system are also of concern, even with generous availability of grants and Medicare/Medicaid incentives (Dixon & Zafar, 2009). What may be practical and effective in a large, urban practice may be impossible to implement in a small, rural clinic.

The development and implementation of Healthcare IT is not currently required of healthcare providers in the United States, but as increasing numbers of providers participate meaningfully in the use of electronic systems, ultimately, adoption of them will become mandatory in a practical sense. As this process unfolds over the next several years, issues of functionality, ethics, and logistics will arise. However, the end results of improved patient safety and reduced healthcare costs will eclipse the initial barriers to Healthcare IT implementation.

References

American Medical Association. (2012). *What is ePrescribing?* Retrieved from http://www.ama-assn.org/ama/pub/eprescribing/what-is-eprescribing.shtml

Centers for Medicare & Medicaid Services. (2012, March 23). 2012: *The year of meaningful use.* Retrieved from http://blog.cms.gov/2012/03/23/2012-the-year-of-meaningful-use/

Consumer-Purchaser Disclosure Project. (2010). *Meaningful use of health information technology: What it is and why it matters to patients and purchasers.* Retrieved from http://www.pbgh.org/storage/documents/commentary/DisclosureMeaningfulUseBackgrounder_03-04-10.pdf

Dixon, B. E. & Zafar, A. (2009). *Inpatient Computerized Provider Order Entry: Findings from the AHRQ Health IT Portfolio* (Prepared by the AHRQ National Resource Center for Health IT). AHRQ Publication

No. 09-0031-EF. Rockville, MD: Agency for Healthcare Research and Quality. Retrieved from http://healthit.ahrq.gov/images/jan09cpoereport/cpoe_issue_paper.htm

Groen, P., Mahootian, F., & Goldstein, D. (2008). *Medical Informatics: Emerging Technologies, 'Open' EHR Systems, and Ethics in the 21st Century*. eBook.

Gutierrez, C. & Scheid, P. (2002). *The history of family medicine and its impact in U.S. health care delivery*. Retrieved from http://www.aafpfoundation.org/online/etc/medialib/found/documents/programs/chfm/foundationgutierrezpaper.Par.0001.File.tmp/foundation-gutierrezpaper.pdf

Hillestad, R. et al. (2012). Can electronic medical record systems transform health care? Potential health benefits, savings, and costs. In L. Shi & D. Singh (Eds.), *Delivering health care in America: A systems approach*. Burlington, MA: Jones & Bartlett.

Miller, R. H. et al. (2012). The value of electronic health records in solo or small group practices. In L. Shi & D. Singh (Eds.), *Delivering health care in America: A systems approach*. Burlington, MA: Jones & Bartlett.

National Academies of Science, Institute of Medicine. (2006). *Preventing medication errors*. Retrieved from http://www.iom.edu/~/media/Files/Report%20Files/2006/Preventing-Medication-Errors-Quality-Chasm-Series/medicationerrorsnew.pdf

National Organization for Research at the University of Chicago (NORC). (2006). *AHRQ 2006 annual patient safety and health information technology conference: Strengthening the connections*. [Conference proceedings]. Washington, D. C.

Shi, L., & Singh, D. (2012). *Delivering health care in America: A systems approach.* Burlington, MA: Jones & Bartlett.

Sutherland, J. (2005). *Regional Health Information Organization (RHIO): Opportunities and risks.* [White Paper]. Retrieved from http://www.himss.org/content/files/sutherland_rhio_whitepaper.pdf

TechTarget. (2010). *Regional Health Information Organization.* Retrieved from http://searchhealthit.techtarget.com/definition/Regional-Health-Information-Organization-RHIO

van der Grinten, P. (2006). *RHIOs aim to transform quality of care and patient safety. Patient Safety and Quality Healthcare*, May/June 2006. Retrieved from http://www.psqh.com/mayjun06/rhio.html

APPENDIX E

Top 200 Drugs

TRADE NAME	Generic Name	*Common Use*
Abilify	aripiprazole	*Anti-Psychotic*
Accupril	quinapril	*Antihypertensive–ACE Inhibitor*
Aciphex	rabeprazole	*Proton Pump Inhibitor*
Actiq	fentanyl	*Analgesic (narcotic–severe pain)*
Actonel	risedronate	*Bisphosphonate (bone resorption inhibitor)*
Actos	pioglitazone	*Anti-Diabetic*
Adderall	amphetamine/dextroamphetamine	*Stimulant (ADHD)*
Adipex	phentermine	*Appetite Suppressant*
Advair	fluticasone/salmeterol	*Asthma/COPD–Bronchodilator /(steroid)*
Advil	ibuprofen	*Analgesic (NSAID)*
Aldactazide	spironolactone/hydrochlorothyazide	*Diuretic Combination*
Aldactone	spironolactone	*Diuretic (potassium-sparing)*
Aleve (OTC)	naproxen	*Analgesic (NSAID)*
Allegra (OTC)	fexofenadine	*Antihistamine*
Alphagan P	brimonidine tartrate	*Alpha Agonist (ophthalmic)*
Altace	ramipril	*Antihypertensive–ACE Inhibitor*
Amaryl	glimepiride	*Anti-Diabetic*
Ambien	zolpidem	*Sleep Aid*

TRADE NAME	Generic Name	*Common Use*
Amoxil	amoxicillin	*Antibiotic (penicillin)*
Antivert	meclizine	*Anti-Vertigo*
Apresoline	hydralazine	*Antihypertensive – Vasodilator*
Aricept	donepezil	*Alzheimer*
Aristospan	triamcinolone	*Corticosteroid*
Arixtra	fonaparinux	*Factor Xa Inhibitor*
Atacand	candesartan	*Antihypertensive–Angiotensin II Receptor Blocker (A2RB)*
Ativan	lorazepam	*Anti-Anxiety/Sedative–Benzodiazepine*
Augmentin	amoxicillin/clavulanate	*Antibiotic (penicillin)*
Avalide	irbesartan/HCTZ	*Antihypertensive–Angiotensin II Receptor Blocker (A2RB)*
Avapro	irbesartan	*Antihypertensive–Angiotensin II Receptor Blocker (A2RB)*
Avelox	moxifloxacin	*Antibiotic (quinolone)*
Avodart	dutasteride	*Prostate Receptor Agonist*
Bactrim	sulfamethoxazole/trimethoprim	*Antibiotic (sulfonamide)*
Bactroban	mupirocin topical	*Anti-Bacterial*
Bayer Aspirin (OTC)	acetylsalicylic acid	*Analgesic NSAID, fever reducer, clot prevention*
Benicar, **Benicar HCT**	olmesartan, olmesartan/hydrochlorothiazide	*Antihypertensive–Angiotensin II Receptor Blocker (A2RB)*
Bentyl	dicyclomine	*Anti-Spasmotic (gastrointestinal)*
Benztropine	benzatropine	*Parkinson Disease*
Biaxin	clarithromycin	*Antibiotic (macrolide)*
Boniva	ibandronate	*Bisphosphonate (bone resorption inhibitor)*
Brilinta	ticagrelor	*Anticoagulant*
Budeprion	bupropion	*Antidepressant*
BuSpar	buspirone	*Anti-Anxiety /Hypnotic*
Byetta	exenatide	*Anti-Diabetic*
Bystolic	nebivolol	*Antihypertensive/Heart Rate Control – Beta Blocker*

TRADE NAME	Generic Name	*Common Use*
Calan	verapamil	*Antihypertensive–Calcium Channel Blocker*
Capoten	captopril	*Antihypertensive–ACE Inhibitor*
Cardizem	diltiazem	*Antihypertensive–Calcium Channel Blocker/ Dysrhythmia*
Cardura	doxazosin	*Antihypertensive–Alpha Receptor Agonist*
Cartia	diltiazem	*Antihypertensive–Calcium Channel Blocker/ Dysrhythmia*
Cataflam	diclofenac	*Analgesic NSAID*
Catapres	clonidine	*Antihypertensive–Alpha Receptor Agonist*
Ceftin	cefuroxime	*Antibiotic (cephalosporin)*
Cefzil	cefprozil	*Antibiotic (cephalosporin)*
Celebrex	celecoxib	*Analgesic NSAID (COX-2 Inhibitor)*
Celexa	citalopram	*Antidepressant*
Chantix	varenicline	*Smoking Cessation*
Cialis	tadalifil	*Erectile Dysfunction*
Cipro	ciprofloxacin	*Antibiotic (quinolone)*
Clarinex	desloratadine	*Antihistamine*
Claritin (OTC)	loratadine	*Antihistamine*
Cleocin	clindamycin	*Antibiotic (macrolide)*
Cogentin	benztropine	*Parkinson Disease*
Colace	docusate sodium	*Stool Softener*
Colchicine	colchicine	*Anti-Gout*
Combivent	albuterol/ipratropium inhaler	*Asthma/COPD–Bronchodilator*
Concerta	methylphenidate	*Stimulant (ADHD)*
Cordarone	amiodarone	*Cardiac dysrhythmia*
Coreg	carvedilol	*Antihypertensive/Heart Rate Control–Beta Blocker*
Cortef	hydrocortisone	*Corticosteroid*
Coumadin	warfarin	*Anticoagulant*
Cozaar	losartan	*Antihypertensive – Angiotensin II Receptor Blocker (A2RB)*
Crestor	rosuvastatin	*Cholesterol Lowering (statin)*
Cymbalta	duloxetine	*Antidepressant*

TRADE NAME	Generic Name	*Common Use*
Daliresp	roflumilast	*COPD*
Demadex	torsemide	*Diuretic*
Depakote / Depakene	divalproex sodium, valproic acid	*Anti-Convulsant/Chronic Pain*
Desyrel	trazodone	*Antidepressant*
Detrol	tolterodine	*Urinary Anti-Spasmotic*
Dexilant	dexlansoprazole	*Proton Pump Inhibitor*
DiaBeta	glyburide	*Anti-Diabetic*
Diflucan	fluconazole	*Anti-Fungal*
Digitek	digoxin	*Cardiac dysrhythmia*
Dilantin	phenytoin	*Anti-Convulsant*
Diovan	valsartan	*Antihypertensive–Angiotensin II Receptor Blocker (A2RB)*
Ditropan	oxybutynin	*Overactive Bladder*
Duragesic	fentanyl transdermal patch	*Analgesic (narcotic)*
Dyrenium	triamterene	*Diuretic (potassium-sparing)*
E.E.S. /Ery-Tab	erythromycin	*Antibiotic (macrolide)*
Edarbi	azilsartan	*Antihypertensive–Angiotensin II Receptor Blocker (A2RB)*
Effexor	venlafaxine	*Antidepressant*
Elavil	amitriptyline	*Depression Pain*
Elidel	pimecrolimus	*Dermatitis Immunosuppressant*
Endocet	oxycodone/acetaminophen	*Analgesic (narcotic)*
Estrace	estradiol	*Estrogen Hormone*
Evista	raloxifene	*Estrogen Modulator*
Feosol	ferrous sulfate	*Iron Deficiency*
Fioricet	butalbital/acetaminophen/ caffeine	*Analgesic (barbiturate)*
Flagyl	metronidazole	*Anti-Microbial*
Flexeril	cyclobenzaprine	*Muscle Relaxant*
Flomax	tamsulosin	*Prostate Receptor Agonist*
Flonase	fluticasone	*Inhaled Steroid*
Folvite	folic acid	*Mineral Supplement*
Fosamax	alendronate	*Bisphosphonate (bone resorption inhibitor)*
Furadantin	nitrofurantoin	*Anti-Microbial*
Glucophage	metformin	*Anti-Diabetic*

TRADE NAME	Generic Name	*Common Use*
Glucotrol	glipizide	*Anti-Diabetic*
Glucovance	metformin/glyburide	*Anti-Diabetic*
Glycolax Laxative	polyethylene glycol	*Laxative*
Horizant	gabapentin enacarbil	*Restless Leg Syndrome*
Humalog Insulin	lispro insulin	*Insulin/Type I Diabetes*
Humulin 70/30	insulin	*Insulin/Type I Diabetes*
Humulin N/Humulin R	insulin	*Insulin/Type I Diabetes*
Hytrin	terazosin	*Antihypertensive–Alpha Receptor Agonist*
Hyzaar	losartan/hydrochlorothiazide	*Antihypertensive–Angiotensin II Receptor Blocker (A2RB) and Diuretic*
Imdur	isosorbide mononitrate	*Nitrate Vasodilator*
Imitrex	sumatriptan	*Seratonin Agonist (Migraine Headache)*
Inderal	propranolol	*Antihypertensive/Heart Rate Control–Beta Blocker*
Indocin	indomethacin	*Analgesic (NSAID)*
Janumet	metformin/sitagliptin	*Anti-Diabetic*
Januvia	sitagliptin	*Anti-Diabetic*
Kadian	morphine sulfate	*Analgesic (narcotic)*
Kay Ciel	potassium chloride powder	*Electrolyte Replacement*
Keflex	cephalexin	*Antibiotic (cephalosporin)*
Kenalog	triamcinolone	*Corticosteroid*
Keppra	levetiracetam	*Anti-Convulsant*
Klonopin	clonazepam	*Anti-Anxiety/Sedative–Benzodiazepine*
K-Lor / K-Dur	potassium chloride	*Electrolyte Replacement*
Klor-Con	potassium chloride	*Electrolyte Replacement*
Lamictal	lamotrigene	*Anti-Convulsant*
Lamisil (OTC)	terbinafine	*Anti-Fungal*
Lanoxin	digoxin	*Inotrope (Heart rate control)*
Lantus	insulin glargine	*Insulin/Type I Diabetes*
Lasix	furosemide	*Diuretic (loop)*
Lescol XL	fluvastatin	*Cholesterol Lowering (statin)*
Levaquin	levofloxacin	*Antibiotic (quinolone)*

TRADE NAME	Generic Name	*Common Use*
Levitra	vardenafil	*Erectile Dysfunction*
Levothroid	levothyroxine	*Hypothyroidism*
Levoxyl	levothyroxine	*Hormone Replacement (thyroid)*
Levsin	hyoscyamine sulfate	*Irritable Bowel*
Lexapro	escitalopram	*Antidepressant*
Lidoderm	lidocaine patch	*Topical Anesthetic*
Lioresal	baclofen	*Muscle Relaxant*
Lipitor	atorvastatin	*Cholesterol Lowering (statin)*
Lodine	etodolac	*Analgesic (NSAID)*
Lomotil	diphenoxylate / atropine	*Antidiarrheal*
Lopid	gemfibrozil	*Cholesterol Lowering*
Lopressor	metoprolol	*Antihypertensive/Heart Rate Control–Beta Blocker*
Lortab	hydrocodone/acetamino-phen	*Analgesic (narcotic)*
Lotensin	benazepril	*Antihypertensive–ACE Inhibitor*
Lotrel	benazepril/amlodipine	*Antihypertensive–ACE Inhibi-tor/Calcium Channel Blocker*
Lotrisone	clotrimazole/betametha-sone	*Anti-Fungal/Steroid*
Lovaza	omega-3/fish oil	*Cholesterol Lowering*
Lozol	indapamide	*Diuretic*
Luminal	phenobarbital	*Anti-Convulsant*
Lunesta	eszopiclone	*Sleep Aid*
Lyrica	pregabalin	*Anti-Convulsant/Neuropathic Pain*
Macrobid	nitrofurantoin	*Anti-Bacterial*
Maxzide	triamterene/hydrochloro-thiazide	*Antihypertensive–Diuretic (potassium-sparing)*
Medrol	methylprednisolone	*Steroid Anti-Inflammatory*
Methadose	methadone	*Opioid Recovery*
Mevacor	lovastatin	*Cholesterol Lowering (statin)*
Miacalcin	calcitonin	*Osteoporosis*
Micronase	glyburide	*Anti-Diabetic*
Microzide	hydrochlorothiazide	*Diuretic (thiazide)*
Minocin	minocycline	*Antibiotic (tetracycline)*
Minocin	nystan	*Anti-Fungal*

TRADE NAME	Generic Name	Common Use
MiraLax (OTC)	polyethylene glycol	*Laxative*
Mobic	meloxicam	*Analgesic NSAID*
Monopril	fosinopril	*Antihypertensive – ACE Inhibitor*
Motrin (OTC)	ibuprofen	*Analgesic NSAID*
MS Contin/MSIR	morphine sulfate	*Analgesic (narcotic)*
Mycostatin	nystatin	*Anti-Fungal*
Namenda	memantine	*Alzheimer*
Naprosyn (OTC)	naproxen sodium	*Analgesic NSAID*
Nasacort	triamcinolone	*Inhaled Steroid*
Nasonex	mometasone	*Nasal Corticosteroid*
Neurontin	gabapentin	*Anti-Convulsant*
Nexium	esomeprazole	*Proton Pump Inhibitor*
Niaspan	niacin	*Cholesterol Lowering*
NitroQuick	nitroglycerin	*Vasodilator*
NitroStat	nitroglycerine	*Vasodilator*
Nizoral	ketoconazole	*Anti-Fungal*
Norco	hydrocodone / acetaminophen	*Analgesic (narcotic)*
Norvasc	amlodipine	*Antihypertensive – Calcium Channel Blocker*
NovoLog	insulin aspart	*Insulin/Type I Diabetes*
Omnicef	cefdinir	*Antibiotic (cephalosporin)*
Oxycontin	oxycodone	*Analgesic (narcotic)*
Pamelor	nortriptyline	*Antidepressant*
Patanol	olopatadine	*Antihistamine*
Paxil	paroxetine	*Antidepressant*
Pepcid (OTC)	famotidine	*Histamine Blocker (H2)*
Percocet	oxycodone/acetaminophen	*Analgesic (narcotic)*
Peridex	chlorhexidine gluconate	*Anti-Microbial/Oral Rinse*
Phenergan	promethazine	*Anti-Nausea*
Phenergan with Codeine	promethazine /codeine	*Cough/Analgesic Supplement*
Plaquenil	hydroxychloroquine	*DMARD Arthritis/Lupus/Malaria*
Plavix	clopidogrel	*Anticoagulant*

TRADE NAME	Generic Name	*Common Use*
Plendil	felodipine	*Antihypertensive–Calcium Channel Blocker*
Pradaxa	dabigatran etexilate	*Anticoagulant*
Pravachol	pravastatin	*Cholesterol Lowering (statin)*
Premarin	conjugated estrogen	*Estrogen Replacement*
Prempro	estrogen/medroxyproges-terone	*Estrogen Replacement*
Prevacid	lansoprazole	*Proton Pump Inhibitor*
Prilosec	omeprazole	*Proton Pump Inhibitor*
Prinivil	lisinopril	*Antihypertensive–ACE Inhibitor*
Prinzide	lisinopril/hydrochlorothia-zide	*Antihypertensive–ACE Inhibi-tor/Diuretic*
Pristiq	desvenlafexine	*Antidepressant*
ProAir	albuterol	*Asthma/COPD–Beta Receptor Agonist–Lungs*
Procardia	nifedipine	*Antihypertensive–Calcium Channel Blocker*
Prometrium	progesterone	*Hormone Replacement*
Proscar	finasteride	*Enzyme Inhibitor (Prostate)*
Protonix	pantoprazole	*Proton Pump Inhibitor*
Proventil	albuterol	*Asthma/COPD–Beta Receptor Agonist-Lungs*
Prozac	fluoxetine	*Antidepressant*
Pulmicort Re-spules	budesonide	*Corticosteroid–Asthma, COPD*
Pyridium	phenazopyridine	*Analgesic (urinary)*
Reglan	metoclopramide	*GI Motility Stimulant*
Relafen	nabumetone	*Analgesic NSAID*
Remeron	mirtazapine	*Antidepressant*
Requip	ropinirole	*Parkinson Disease*
Restoril	temazepam	*Sleep Aid (Benzodiazepine)*
Rheumatrex	methotrexate	*Anti-Rheumatic (DMARD)*
Rhinocort Aqua	budesonide	*Corticosteroid*
Risperdal	risperidone	*Anti-Psychotic*
Ritalin	methylphenidate	*ADHD--stimulant*
Robaxin	methocarbamol	*Muscle Relaxant*
Robitussin	cheritussin	*Cold/Cough Syrup*

TRADE NAME	Generic Name	*Common Use*
Roxicet	oxycodone and acetaminophen	*Analgesic (narcotic)*
Septra	sulfamethoxazole/trimethoprim	*Antibiotic (sulfonamide)*
Septra	sulfamethoxazole/trimethoprim	*Antibiotic (sulfonamide)*
Serevent Diskus	salmeterol	*Asthma/COPD*
Seroquel	quetiapine	*Anti-Psychotic*
Sinemet	carbidopa/levodopa	*Anti-Parkinson*
Sinequan	doxepin	*Antidepressant*
Singulair	montelukast	*Leukotriene Inhibitor (Allergies)*
Skelaxin	metaxalone	*Muscle Relaxant*
SMZ-TMP (also Bactrim, Septra)	sulfamethoxazole/trimethoprim	*Antibiotic (sulfonamide)*
Solu-Medrol	methylprednisolone	*Corticosteroid*
Soma	carisoprodol	*Muscle Relaxant*
Spiriva	tiotropium	*COPD*
Sterapred	prednisone	*Corticosteroid*
Strattera	atomoxetine	*Norepinephrine Reuptake Inhibitor (ADHD)*
Sublimaze / Actiq	fentanyl	*Analgesic (narcotic)*
Suboxone	buprenorphine	*Opioid Recovery*
Synthroid	levothyroxine	*Hormone Replacement*
Tamiflu	oseltamivir	*Anti-Viral (Flu)*
Tamofen	tamoxifen citrate	*Antineoplastic Agent*
Tegretol	carbamazepine	*Anti-Convulsant*
Temovate	clobetasol	*Corticosteroid*
Tenoretic	atenolol/chlorthalidone	*Antihypertensive/Heart Rate Control–Beta Blocker)/Diuretic*
Tenormin	atenolol	*Antihypertensive/Heart Rate Control–Beta Blocker*
Tessalon Perles	benzonatate	*Cough Suppressant*
Theo-Dur	theophylline	*Asthma/COPD*
Tiazac	diltiazem	*Antihypertensive–Calcium Channel Blocker/Dysrhythmia*
Timoptic / Blocadren	timolol maleate	*Alpha Agonist, ophthalmic*

TRADE NAME	Generic Name	*Common Use*
TobraDex	tobramycin/dexamethasone	*Ocular antibiotic/corticosteroid*
Topamax	topiramate	*Anti-Convulsant*
Toprol	metoprolol	*Antihypertensive/Heart Rate Control–Beta Blocker*
Tradjenta	linagliptin	*Anti-Diabetic*
Trandate	labetalol	*Antihypertensive–Alpha & Beta Blocker*
Trexall	methotrexate	*Antineoplastic Agent*
Tricor	fenofibrate	*Cholesterol Lowering*
Trileptal	oxcarbazepine	*Anti-Convulsant*
Trimox	amoxicillin	*Antibiotic (penicillin)*
Tussionex	hydrocodone/chlorpheniramine	*Narcotic/Antihistamine*
Tylenol No. 3	codeine/acetaminophen	*Analgesic (narcotic)*
Uloric	febuxostat	*Gout*
Ultracet	tramadol/acetaminophen	*Analgesic (non-narcotic)*
Ultram	tramadol	*Analgesic (non-narcotic)*
Valium	diazepam	*Anti-Anxiety/Sedative–Benzodiazepine*
Valtrex	valacyclovir	*Anti-Viral*
Vasotec	enalapril	*Antihypertensive–ACE Inhibitor*
Ventolin	albuterol	*Asthma/COPD–Bronchodilator*
Verelan	verapamil	*Antihypertensive–Calcium Channel Blocker*
Viagra	sildenafil	*Erectile Dysfunction*
Vibramycin	doxycycline	*Antibiotic (tetracycline)*
Vicodin	hydrocodone/acetaminophen	*Analgesic (narcotic)*
Vicodin	hydrocodone/acetaminophen	*Analgesic (narcotic)*
Vigamox	moxifloxacin	*Antibiotic (quinolone)*
Viibryd	vilazodone	*Antidepressant*
Vistaril	hydroxyzine	*Antihistamine*
Vivelle-Dot	estradiol	*Hormone Replacement*
Voltaren	diclofenac sodium	*Analgesic (NSAID)*
VoSpire	albuterol	*Asthma COPD*

TRADE NAME	Generic Name	*Common Use*
Vytorin	ezetimibe/simvastatin	*Cholesterol Lowering Combination*
Vyvanse	lisdexamfetamine	*Stimulant (ADHD)*
Wellbutrin	bupropion	*Antidepressant*
Xalatan	latanoprost	*Ophthalmic Prostaglandin*
Xanax	alprazolam	*Anti-Anxiety/Sedative–Benzodiazepine*
Xopenex	levalbuterol	*Asthma/COPD*
Zanaflex	tizanidine	*Multiple Sclerosis*
Zantac (OTC)	ranitidine	*Histamine Blocker (H2)*
Zebeta	bisoprolol	*Antihypertensive/Heart Rate Control–Beta Blocker*
Zestoretic	lisinopril/hydrochlorothiazide	*Antihypertensive–ACE Inhibitor/Diuretic*
Zestril	lisinopril	*Antihypertensive–ACE Inhibitor*
Zetia	ezetimibe	*Cholesterol Lowering*
Ziac	bisoprolol/hydrochlorothiazide	*Antihypertensive–Beta Blocker/ Diuretic*
Zithromax	azithromycin	*Antibiotic (macrolide)*
Zocor	simvastatin	*Cholesterol Lowering (statin)*
Zofran	ondansetron	*Anti-Nausea*
Zoloft	sertraline	*Antidepressant*
Zovirax	acyclovir	*Anti-Viral*
Zyloprim	allopurinol	*Gout*
Zyprexa	olanzapine	*Anti-Psychotic*
Zyrtec	Cetirizine	*Antihistamine*

Note that in this list, generic names are not capitalized. Many references now list the generic name with a capital letter, or use all caps for both names, which can lead to confusion. Please review both names for all your medications to assure there are no duplications.

This list is certainly not all-inclusive of medications prescribed, and new approvals are issued every month. Centerwatch (*http://www.centerwatch.com/*) keeps a list of FDA approvals, so new medications can be reviewed at this website.

ABOUT THE AUTHOR

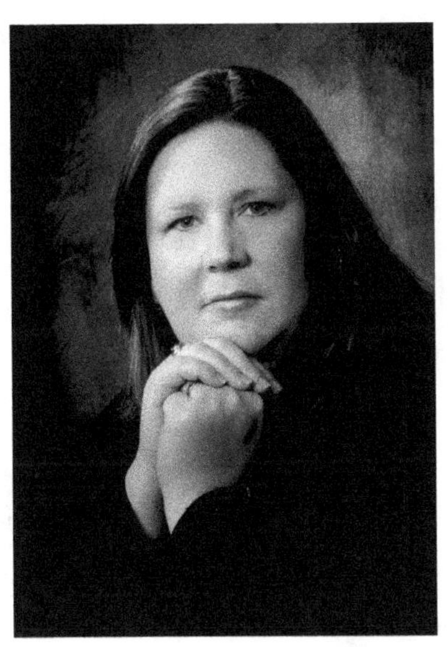

Val grew up in a small West Texas town, where looking after family and neighbors was part of life. Having spent her entire adult career in medicine of some sort, helping her parents with medical issues started when her father had a heart attack at the age of 41. She remembers her mother's surprise as she explained the procedure and goals of his upcoming bypass surgery, knowing her parents had thought that being a paramedic just meant a big white ambulance and very few holidays at home. Knowing this information about his surgery was comforting, but more specifically, the explanation was in their language, not the technical medical jargon the surgeon had used.

Being able to teach someone about how their body is supposed to function, then what is not working right to cause a condition or disease, has been one of Val's passions. Education is an important part of improving healthcare. But new knowledge had to be shared at a level the learner could understand, whether teaching to a patient or a physician.

Val has taught in emergency medicine for years, in Emergency Medical Technician and Paramedic courses, Basic and Advanced Cardiac Life Support courses, Basic Trauma Life Support courses, and others. When it came time to retire from being a paramedic, her desire to help didn't slow, so she obtained her Bachelor of Science in Nursing from West Texas A&M University in Canyon, then began working again with patients, teaching and healing. During this time in her life, her father's health began to decline, and some of the lessons she learned about advocating for a family member were the impetus for this book.

ABOUT THE ILLUSTRATOR

Cary Raulston studied Commercial Art at Texas State Technical Institute in Amarillo, TX. He does a weekly cartoon strip for the Panhandle Progress, as well as freelance art. cbear_2k@yahoo.com

www.ingramcontent.com/pod-product-compliance
Lightning Source LLC
Chambersburg PA
CBHW070755290326
41931CB00011BA/2018
9780985418014